FASTING FOR BEGINNERS

FASTING SECRETS **REVEALED**

Say Goodbye to Belly Fat With Intermittent Fasting

CARLO DIXON

Copyright © 2020 Carlo Dixon

All Rights Reserved

Copyright 2020 By Carlo Dixon - All rights reserved.

The following book is produced below with the goal of providing information that is as accurate and reliable as possible. Regardless, purchasing this book can be seen as consent to the fact that both the publisher and the author of this book are in no way experts on the topics discussed within and that any recommendations or suggestions that are made herein are for entertainment purposes only. Professionals should be consulted as needed prior to undertaking any of the action endorsed herein.

This declaration is deemed fair and valid by both the American Bar Association and the Committee of Publishers Association and is legally binding throughout the United States.

Furthermore, the transmission, duplication or reproduction of any of the following work including specific information will be considered an illegal act irrespective of if it is done electronically or in print. This extends to creating a secondary or tertiary copy of the work or a recorded copy and is only allowed with express written consent from the Publisher. All additional right reserved.

The information in the following pages is broadly considered to be a truthful and accurate account of facts and as such any inattention, use or misuse of the information in question by the reader will render any resulting actions solely under their purview. There are no scenarios in which the publisher or the original author of this work can be in any fashion deemed liable for any hardship or damages that may befall them after undertaking information described herein.

Additionally, the information in the following pages is intended only for informational purposes and should thus be thought of as universal. As befitting its nature, it is presented without assurance regarding its prolonged validity or interim quality. Trademarks that are mentioned are done without written consent and can in no way be considered an endorsement from the trademark holder.

Table of Contents

PART I

Smoothie Diet Recipes

The smoothie diet is all about replacing some of your meals with smoothies that are loaded with veggies and fruits. It has been found that the smoothie diet is very helpful in losing weight along with excess fat. The ingredients of the smoothies will vary, but they will focus mainly on vegetables and fruits. The best part about the smoothie diet is that there is no need to count your calorie intake and less food tracking. The diet is very low in calories and is also loaded with phytonutrients.

Apart from weight loss, there are various other benefits of the smoothie diet. It can help you to stay full for a longer time as most smoothies are rich in fiber. It can also help you to control your cravings as smoothies are full of flavor and nutrients. Whenever you feel like snacking, just prepare a smoothie, and you are good to go. Also, smoothies can aid in digestion as they are rich in important minerals and vitamins. Fruits such as mango are rich in carotenoids that can help in improving your skin quality. As the smoothie diet is mainly based on veggies and fruits, it can detoxify your body.

In this section, you will find various recipes of smoothies that you can include in your smoothie diet.

Chapter 1: Fruit Smoothies

The best way of having fruits is by making smoothies. Fruit smoothies can help you start your day with loads of nutrients so that you can remain energetic throughout the day. Here are some easy-to-make fruit smoothie recipes that you can enjoy during any time of the day.

Quick Fruit Smoothie

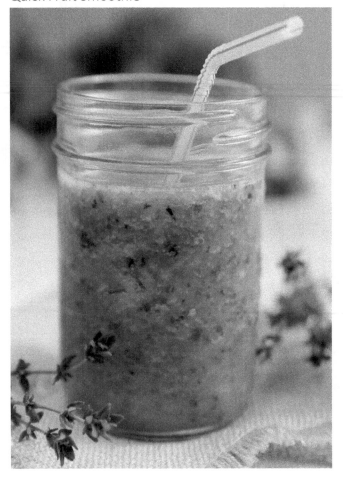

Total Prep & Cooking Time: Fifteen minutes

Yields: Four servings

Nutrition Facts: Calories: 115.2 | Protein: 1.2g | Carbs: 27.2g | Fat: 0.5g | Fiber: 3.6g

Ingredients

- One cup of strawberries
- One banana (cut in chunks)
- Two peaches
- Two cups of ice
- One cup of orange and mango juice

Method:

1. Add banana, strawberries, and peaches in a blender.

2. Blend until frothy and smooth.

3. Add the orange and mango juice and blend again. Add ice for adjusting the consistency and blend for two minutes.

4. Divide the smoothie in glasses and serve with mango chunks from the top.

Triple Threat Smoothie

Total Prep & Cooking Time: Ten minutes

Yields: Four servings

Nutrition Facts: Calories: 132.2 | Protein: 3.4g | Carbs: 27.6g | Fat: 1.3g | Fiber: 2.7g

Ingredients

- One kiwi (sliced)
- One banana (chopped)
- One cup of each
  - Ice cubes
  - Strawberries
- Half cup of blueberries
- One-third cup of orange juice
- Eight ounces of peach yogurt

Method:

1. Add kiwi, strawberries, and bananas in a food processor.

2. Blend until smooth.

3. Add the blueberries along with orange juice. Blend again for two minutes.

4. Add peach yogurt and ice cubes. Give it a pulse.

5. Pour the prepared smoothie in smoothie glasses and serve with blueberry chunks from the top.

Tropical Smoothie

Total Prep & Cooking Time: Fifteen minutes

Yields: Two servings

Nutrition Facts: Calories: 127.3 | Protein: 1.6g | Carbs: 30.5g | Fat: 0.7g | Fiber: 4.2g

Ingredients

- One mango (seeded)
- One papaya (cubed)
- Half cup of strawberries
- One-third cup of orange juice
- Five ice cubes

Method:

1. Add mango, strawberries, and papaya in a blender. Blend the ingredients until smooth.

2. Add ice cubes and orange juice for adjusting the consistency.

3. Blend again.

4. Serve with strawberry chunks from the top.

Fruit and Mint Smoothie

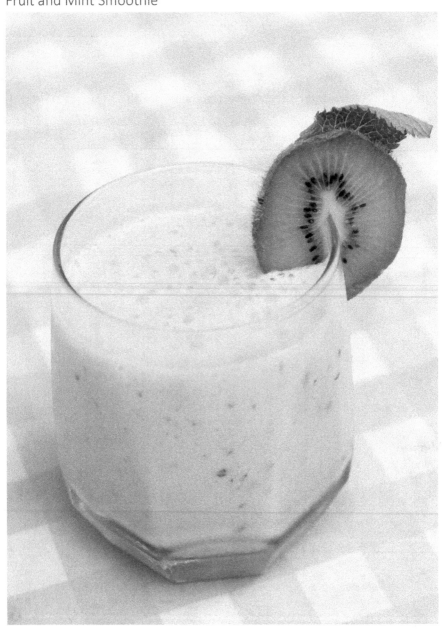

Total Prep & Cooking Time: Fifteen minutes

Yields: Two servings

Nutrition Facts: Calories: 90.3 | Protein: 0.7g | Carbs: 21.4g | Fat: 0.4g | Fiber: 2.5g

Ingredients

- One-fourth cup of each
    - Applesauce (unsweetened)
    - Red grapes (seedless, frozen)
- One tbsp. of lime juice
- Three strawberries (frozen)
- One cup of pineapple cubes
- Three mint leaves

Method:

1. Add grapes, lime juice, and applesauce in a blender. Blend the ingredients until frothy and smooth.

2. Add pineapple cubes, mint leaves, and frozen strawberries in the blender. Pulse the ingredients for a few times until the pineapple and strawberries are crushed.

3. Serve with mint leaves from the top.

Banana Smoothie

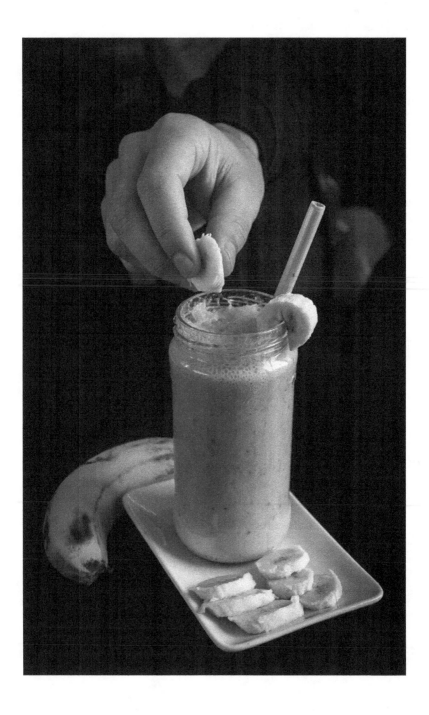

Total Prep & Cooking Time: Ten minutes

Yields: Four servings

Nutrition Facts: Calories: 122.6 | Protein: 1.3g | Carbs: 34.6g | Fat: 0.4g | Fiber: 2.2g

Ingredients

- Three bananas (sliced)
- One cup of fresh pineapple juice
- One tbsp. of honey
- Eight cubes of ice

Method:

1. Combine the bananas and pineapple juice in a blender.

2. Blend until smooth.

3. Add ice cubes along with honey.

4. Blend for two minutes.

5. Serve immediately.

Dragon Fruit Smoothie

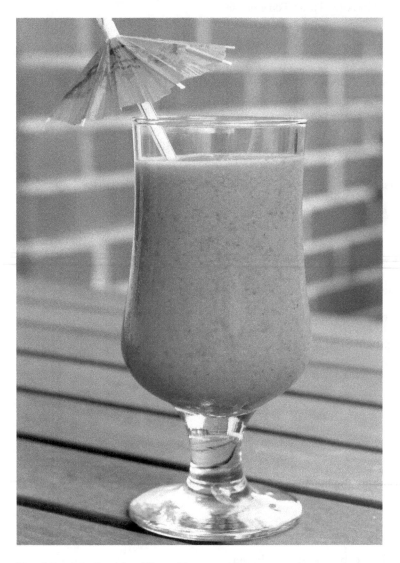

Total Prep & Cooking Time: Twenty minutes

Yields: Four servings

Nutrition Facts: Calories: 147.6 | Protein: 5.2g | Carbs: 21.4g | Fat: 6.4g | Fiber: 2.9g

Ingredients

- One-fourth cup of almonds
- Two tbsps. of shredded coconut
- One tsp. of chocolate chips
- One cup of yogurt
- One dragon fruit (chopped)
- Half cup of pineapple cubes
- One tbsp. of honey

Method:

1. Add almonds, dragon fruit, coconut, and chocolate chips in a high power blender. Blend until smooth.

2. Add yogurt, pineapple, and honey. Blend well.

3. Serve with chunks of dragon fruit from the top.

Kefir Blueberry Smoothie

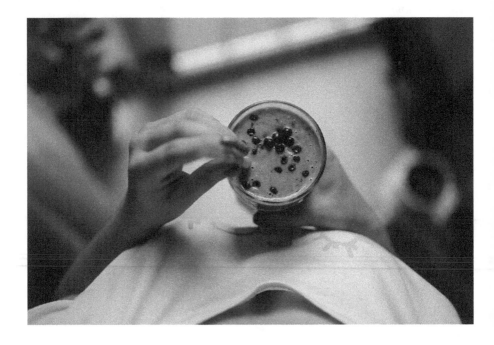

Total Prep & Cooking Time: Fifteen minutes

Yields: Two servings

Nutrition Facts: Calories: 304.2 | Protein: 7.3g | Carbs: 41.3g | Fat: 13.2g | Fiber: 4.6g

Ingredients

- Half cup of kefir
- One cup of blueberries (frozen)
- Half banana (cubed)

- One tbsp. of almond butter
- Two tsps. of honey

Method:

1. Add blueberries, banana cubes, and kefir in a blender.

2. Blend until smooth.

3. Add honey and almond butter.

4. Pulse the smoothie for a few times.

5. Serve immediately.

Ginger Fruit Smoothie

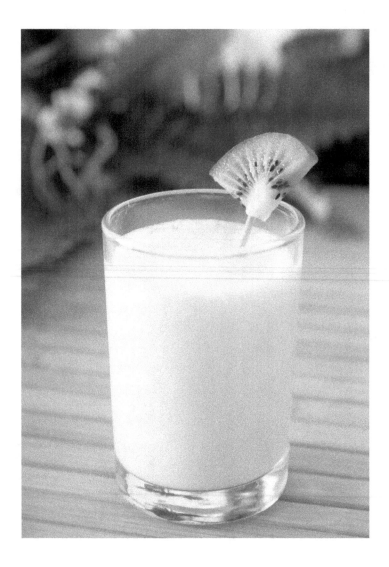

Total Prep & Cooking Time: Fifteen minutes

Yields: Two servings

Nutrition Facts: Calories: 160.2 | Protein: 1.9g | Carbs: 41.3g | Fat: 0.7g | Fiber: 5.6g

Ingredients

- One-fourth cup of each
    - Blueberries (frozen)
    - Green grapes (seedless)
- Half cup of green apple (chopped)
- One cup of water
- Three strawberries
- One piece of ginger
- One tbsp. of agave nectar

Method:

1. Add blueberries, grapes, and water in a blender. Blend the ingredients.

2. Add green apple, strawberries, agave nectar, and ginger. Blend for making thick slushy.

3. Serve immediately.

Fruit Batido

Total Prep & Cooking Time: Fifteen minutes

Yields: Six servings

Nutrition Facts: Calories: 129.3 | Protein: 4.2g | Carbs: 17.6g | Fat: 4.6g | Fiber: 0.6g

Ingredients

- One can of evaporated milk
- One cup of papaya (chopped)
- One-fourth cup of white sugar
- One tsp. of vanilla extract
- One tsp. of cinnamon (ground)
- One tray of ice cubes

Method:

1. Add papaya, white sugar, cinnamon, and vanilla extract in a food processor. Blend the ingredients until smooth.

2. Add milk and ice cubes. Blend for making slushy.

3. Serve immediately.

Banana Peanut Butter Smoothie
Total Prep & Cooking Time: Ten minutes

Yields: Four servings

Nutrition Facts: Calories: 332 | Protein: 13.2g | Carbs: 35.3g | Fat: 17.8g |
Fiber: 3.9g

Ingredients

- Two bananas (cubed)
- Two cups of milk
- Half cup of peanut butter
- Two tbsps. of honey
- Two cups of ice cubes

Method:

1. Add banana cubes and peanut butter in a blender. Blend for making a smooth paste.

2. Add milk, ice cubes, and honey. Blend the ingredients until smooth.

3. Serve with banana chunks from the top.

Chapter 2: Breakfast Smoothies

Smoothie forms an essential part of breakfast in the smoothie diet plan. Here are some breakfast smoothie recipes for you that can be included in your daily breakfast plan.

Berry Banana Smoothie

Total Prep & Cooking Time: Twenty minutes

Yields: Two servings

Nutrition Facts: Calories: 330 | Protein: 6.7g | Carbs: 56.3g | Fat: 13.2g | Fiber: 5.5g

Ingredients

- One cup of each
  - Strawberries
  - Peaches (cubed)
  - Apples (cubed)
- One banana (cubed)
- Two cups of vanilla ice cream
- Half cup of ice cubes
- One-third cup of milk

Method:

1. Place strawberries, peaches, banana, and apples in a blender. Pulse the ingredients.

2. Add milk, ice cream, and ice cubes. Blend the smoothie until frothy and smooth.

3. Serve with a scoop of ice cream from the top.

Berry Surprise

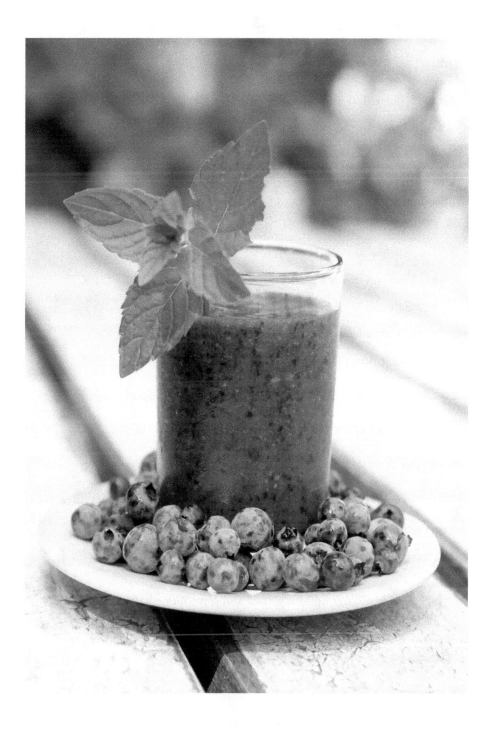

Total Prep & Cooking Time: Ten minutes

Yields: Two servings

Nutrition Facts: Calories: 164.2 | Protein: 1.2g | Carbs: 40.2g | Fat: 0.4g | Fiber: 4.8g

Ingredients

- One cup of strawberries
- Half cup of pineapple cubes
- One-third cup of raspberries
- Two tbsps. of limeade concentrate (frozen)

Method:

1. Combine pineapple cubes, strawberries, and raspberries in a food processor. Blend the ingredients until smooth.

2. Add the frozen limeade and blend again.

3. Divide the smoothie in glasses and serve immediately.

Coconut Matcha Smoothie

Total Prep & Cooking Time: Twenty minutes

Yields: Two servings

Nutrition Facts: Calories: 362 | Protein: 7.2g | Carbs: 70.1g | Fat: 8.7g | Fiber: 12.1g

Ingredients

- One large banana
- One cup of frozen mango cubes
- Two leaves of kale (torn)
- Three tbsps. of white beans (drained)
- Two tbsps. of shredded coconut (unsweetened)
- Half tsp. of matcha green tea (powder)
- Half cup of water

Method:

1. Add cubes of mango, banana, white beans, and kale in a blender. Blend all the ingredients until frothy and smooth.

2. Add shredded coconut, white beans, water, and green tea powder. Blend for thirty seconds.

3. Serve with shredded coconut from the top.

Cantaloupe Frenzy

Total Prep & Cooking Time: Ten minutes

Yields: Three servings

Nutrition Facts: Calories: 108.3 | Protein: 1.6g | Carbs: 26.2g | Fat: 0.2g | Fiber: 1.6g

Ingredients

- One cantaloupe (seeded, chopped)
- Three tbsps. of white sugar
- Two cups of ice cubes

Method:

1. Place the chopped cantaloupe along with white sugar in a blender. Puree the mixture.

2. Add cubes of ice and blend again.

3. Pour the smoothie in serving glasses. Serve immediately.

Berry Lemon Smoothie

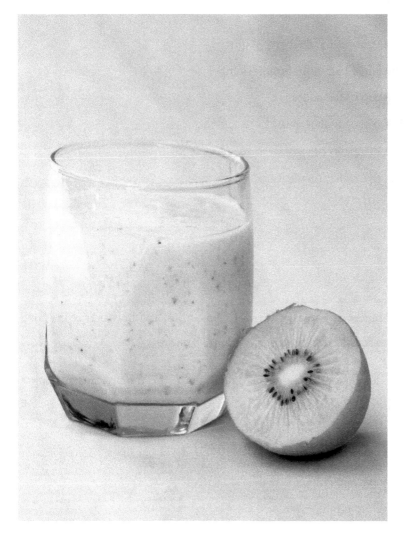

Total Prep & Cooking Time: Ten minutes

Yields: Four servings

Nutrition Facts: Calories: 97.2 | Protein: 5.4g | Carbs: 19.4g | Fat: 0.4g | Fiber: 1.8g

Ingredients

- Eight ounces of blueberry yogurt
- One and a half cup of milk (skim)
- One cup of ice cubes
- Half cup of blueberries
- One-third cup of strawberries
- One tsp. of lemonade mix

Method:

1. Add blueberry yogurt, skim milk, blueberries, and strawberries in a food processor. Blend the ingredients until smooth.

2. Add lemonade mix and ice cubes. Pulse the mixture for making a creamy and smooth smoothie.

3. Divide the smoothie in glasses and serve.

Orange Glorious

Total Prep & Cooking Time: Ten minutes

Yields: Four servings

Nutrition Facts: Calories: 212 | Protein: 3.4g | Carbs: 47.3g | Fat: 1.5g | Fiber: 0.5g

Ingredients

- Six ounces of orange juice concentrate (frozen)
- One cup of each
  - Water
  - Milk
- Half cup of white sugar
- Twelve ice cubes
- One tsp. of vanilla extract

Method:

1. Combine orange juice concentrate, white sugar, milk, and water in a blender.

2. Add vanilla extract and ice cubes. Blend the mixture until smooth.

3. Pour the smoothie in glasses and enjoy!

Grapefruit Smoothie

Total Prep & Cooking Time: Ten minutes

Yields: Two servings

Nutrition Facts: Calories: 200.3 | Protein: 4.7g | Carbs: 46.3g | Fat: 1.2g | Fiber: 7.6g

Ingredients

- Three grapefruits (peeled)
- One cup of water
- Three ounces of spinach
- Six ice cubes
- Half-inch piece of ginger
- One tsp. of flax seeds

Method:

1. Combine spinach, grapefruit, and ginger in a high power blender. Blend until smooth.

2. Add water, flax seeds, and ice cubes. Blend smooth.

3. Pour the smoothie in glasses and serve.

Sour Smoothie

Total Prep & Cooking Time: Ten minutes

Yields: Two servings

Nutrition Facts: Calories: 102.6 | Protein: 2.3g | Carbs: 30.2g | Fat: 0.7g | Fiber: 7.9g

Ingredients

- One cup of ice cubes
- Two fruit limes (peeled)
- One orange (peeled)
- One lemon (peeled)
- One kiwi (peeled)
- One tsp. of honey

Method:

1. Add fruit limes, lemon, orange, and kiwi in a food processor. Blend until frothy and smooth.

2. Add cubes of ice and honey. Pulse the ingredients.

3. Divide the smoothie in glasses and enjoy!

Ginger Orange Smoothie

Total Prep & Cooking Time: Ten minutes

Yields: One serving

Nutrition Facts: Calories: 115.6 | Protein: 2.2g | Carbs: 27.6g | Fat: 1.3g | Fiber: 5.7g

Ingredients

- One large orange
- Two carrots (peeled, cut in chunks)
- Half cup of each
  - Red grapes
  - Ice cubes
- One-fourth cup of water
- One-inch piece of ginger

Method:

1. Combine carrots, grapes, and orange in a high power blender. Blend until frothy and smooth.

2. Add ice cubes, ginger, and water. Blend the ingredients for thirty seconds.

3. Serve immediately.

Cranberry Smoothie

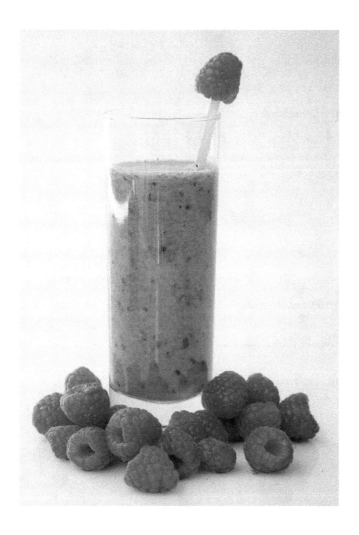

Total Prep & Cooking Time: One hour and ten minutes

Yields: Two servings

Nutrition Facts: Calories: 155.9 | Protein: 2.2g | Carbs: 33.8g | Fat: 1.6g | Fiber: 5.2g

Ingredients

- One cup of almond milk
- Half cup of mixed berries (frozen)
- One-third cup of cranberries
- One banana

Method:

1. Blend mixed berries, banana, and cranberries in a high power food processor. Blend until smooth.

2. Add almond milk and blend again for twenty seconds.

3. Refrigerate the prepared smoothie for one hour.

4. Serve chilled.

Creamsicle Smoothie

Total Prep & Cooking Time: Ten minutes

Yields: Two servings

Nutrition Facts: Calories: 121.3 | Protein: 4.7g | Carbs: 19.8g | Fat: 2.5g | Fiber: 0.3g

Ingredients

- One cup of orange juice
- One and a half cup of crushed ice
- Half cup of milk
- One tsp. of white sugar

Method:

1. Blend milk, orange juice, white sugar, and ice in a high power blender.

2. Keep blending until there is no large chunk of ice. Try to keep the consistency of slushy.

3. Serve immediately.

Sunshine Smoothie

Total Prep & Cooking Time: Thirty minutes

Yields: Four servings

Nutrition Facts: Calories: 176.8 | Protein: 4.2g | Carbs: 39.9g | Fat: 1.3g | Fiber: 3.9g

Ingredients

- Two nectarines (pitted, quartered)
- One banana (cut in chunks)
- One orange (peeled, quartered)
- One cup of vanilla yogurt
- One-third cup of orange juice
- One tbsp. of honey

Method:

1. Add banana chunks, nectarines, and orange in a blender. Blender for two minutes.

2. Add vanilla yogurt, honey, and orange juice. Blend the ingredients until frothy and smooth.

3. Pour the smoothie in glasses and serve.

Chapter 3: Vegetable Smoothies

Apart from fruit smoothies, vegetable smoothies can also provide you with essential nutrients. In fact, vegetable smoothies are tasty as well. So, here are some vegetable smoothie recipes for you.

Mango Kale Berry Smoothie
Total Prep & Cooking Time: Ten minutes

Yields: Four servings

Nutrition Facts: Calories: 117.3 | Protein: 3.1g | Carbs: 22.6g | Fat: 3.6g | Fiber: 6.2g

Ingredients

- One cup of orange juice
- One-third cup of kale
- One and a half cup of mixed berries (frozen)
- Half cup of mango chunks
- One-fourth cup of water
- Two tbsps. of chia seeds

Method:

1. Take a high power blender and add kale, orange juice, berries, mango chunks, chia seeds, and half a cup of water.

2. Blend the ingredients on high settings until smooth.

3. In case the smoothie is very thick, you can adjust the consistency by adding more water.

4. Pour the smoothie in glasses and serve.

Breakfast Pink Smoothie

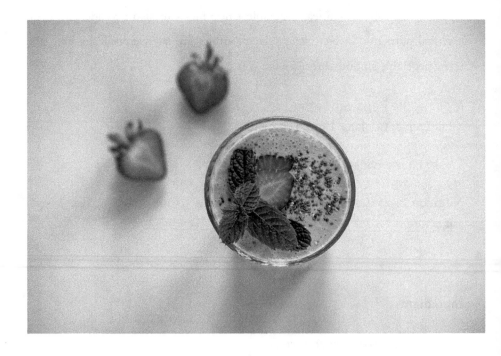

Total Prep & Cooking Time: Ten minutes

Yields: Two servings

Nutrition Facts: Calories: 198.3 | Protein: 12.3g | Carbs: 6.3g | Fat: 4.5g | Fiber: 8.8g

Ingredients

- One and a half cup of strawberries (frozen)
- One cup of raspberries
- One orange (peeled)

- Two carrots
- Two cups of coconut milk (light)
- One small beet (quartered)

Method:

1. Add strawberries, raspberries, and orange in a blender. Blend until frothy and smooth.

2. Add beet, carrots, and coconut milk.

3. Blend again for one minute.

4. Divide the smoothie in glasses and serve.

Butternut Squash Smoothie

Total Prep & Cooking Time: Five minutes

Yields: Four servings

Nutrition Facts: Calories: 127.3 | Protein: 2.3g | Carbs: 32.1g | Fat: 1.2g | Fiber: 0.6g

Ingredients

- Two cups of almond milk
- One-fourth cup of nut butter (of your choice)
- One cup of water
- One and a half cup of butternut squash (frozen)
- Two ripe bananas
- One tsp. of cinnamon (ground)
- Two tbsps. of hemp protein
- Half cup of strawberries
- One tbsp. of chia seeds
- Half tbsp. of bee pollen

Method:

1. Add butternut squash, bananas, strawberries, and almond milk in a blender. Blend until frothy and smooth.

2. Add water, nut butter, cinnamon, hemp protein, chia seeds, and bee pollen. Blend the ingredients f0r two minutes.

3. Divide the smoothie in glasses and enjoy!

Zucchini and Wild Blueberry Smoothie

Total Prep & Cooking Time: Ten minutes

Yields: Three servings

Nutrition Facts: Calories: 190.2 | Protein: 7.3g | Carbs: 27.6g | Fat: 8.1g | Fiber: 5.7g

Ingredients

- One banana
- One cup of wild blueberries (frozen)
- One-fourth cup of peas (frozen)
- Half cup of zucchini (frozen, chopped)
- One tbsp. of each
  - Hemp hearts
  - Chia seeds
  - Bee pollen
- One-third cup of almond milk
- Two tbsps. of nut butter (of your choice)
- Ten cubes of ice

Method:

1. Add blueberries, banana, peas, and zucchini in a high power blender. Blend the ingredients for two minutes.

2. Add chia seeds, hemp hearts, almond milk, bee pollen, nut butter, and ice. Blend the mixture for making a thick and smooth smoothie.

3. Pour the smoothie in glasses and serve with chopped blueberries from the top.

Cauliflower and Blueberry Smoothie

Total Prep & Cooking Time: Five minutes

Yields: Two servings

Nutrition Facts: Calories: 201.9 | Protein: 7.1g | Carbs: 32.9g | Fat: 10.3g | Fiber: 4.6g

Ingredients

- One Clementine (peeled)
- Three-fourth cup of cauliflower (frozen)
- Half cup of wild blueberries (frozen)
- One cup of Greek yogurt
- One tbsp. of peanut butter
- Bunch of spinach

Method:

1. Add cauliflower, Clementine, and blueberries in a blender. Blend for one minute.

2. Add peanut butter, spinach, and yogurt. Pulse the ingredients for two minutes until smooth.

3. Divide the prepared smoothie in glasses and enjoy!

Immunity Booster Smoothie

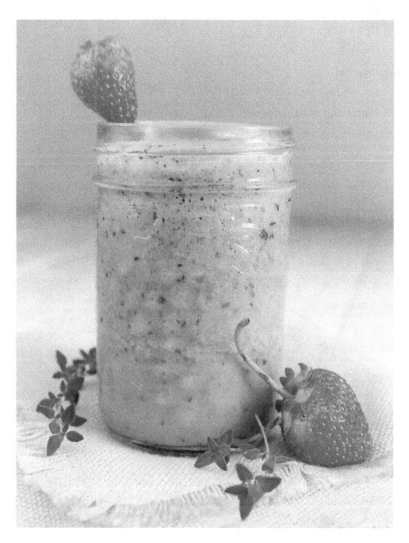

Total Prep & Cooking Time: Ten minutes

Yields: Two servings

Nutrition Facts: Calories: 301.9 | Protein: 5.4g | Carbs: 70.7g | Fat: 4.3g | Fiber: 8.9g

Ingredients

For the orange layer:

- One persimmon (quartered)
- One ripe mango (chopped)
- One lime (juiced)
- One tbsp. of nut butter (of your choice)
- Half tsp. of turmeric powder
- One pinch of cayenne pepper
- One cup of coconut milk

For the pink layer:

- One small beet (cubed)
- One cup of berries (frozen)
- One pink grapefruit (quartered)
- One-fourth cup of pomegranate juice
- Half cup of water
- Six leaves of mint
- One tsp. of honey

Method:

1. Add the ingredients for the orange layer in a blender. Blend for making a smooth liquid.

2. Pour the orange liquid evenly in serving glasses.

3. Add the pink layer ingredients in a blender. Blend for making a smooth liquid.

4. Pour the pink liquid slowly over the orange layer.

5. Pour in such a way so that both layers can be differentiated.

6. Serve immediately.

Ginger, Carrot, and Turmeric Smoothie

Total Prep & Cooking Time: Forty minutes

Yields: Two servings

Nutrition Facts: Calories: 140 | Protein: 2.6g | Carbs: 30.2g | Fat: 2.2g | Fiber: 5.6g

Ingredients

For carrot juice:

- Two cups of water
- Two and a half cups of carrots

For smoothie:

- One ripe banana (sliced)
- One cup of pineapple (frozen, cubed)
- Half tbsp. of ginger
- One-fourth tsp. of turmeric (ground)
- Half cup of carrot juice
- One tbsp. of lemon juice
- One-third cup of almond milk

Method:

1. Add water and carrots in a high power blender. Blend on high settings for making smooth juice.

2. Take a dish towel and strain the juice over a bowl. Squeeze the towel for taking out most of the juice.

3. Add the ingredients for the smoothie in a blender and blend until frothy and creamy.

4. Add carrot juice and blend again.

5. Pour the smoothie in glasses and serve.

Romaine Mango Smoothie

Total Prep & Cooking Time: Five minutes

Yields: Two servings

Nutrition Facts: Calories: 117.3 | Protein: 2.6g | Carbs: 30.2g | Fat: 0.9g | Fiber: 4.2g

Ingredients

- Sixteen ounces of coconut water
- Two mangoes (pitted)
- One head of romaine (chopped)
- One banana
- One orange (peeled)
- Two cups of ice

Method:

1. Add mango, romaine, orange, and banana in a high power blender. Blend the ingredients until frothy and smooth.

2. Add coconut water and ice cubes. Blend for one minute.

3. Pour the prepared smoothie in glasses and serve.

Fig Zucchini Smoothie
Total Prep & Cooking Time: Ten minutes

Yields: Two servings

Nutrition Facts: Calories: 243.3 | Protein: 14.4g | Carbs: 74.3g | Fat: 27.6g | Fiber: 9.3g

Ingredients

- Half cup of cashew nuts
- One tsp. of cinnamon (ground)
- Two figs (halved)
- One banana
- Half tsp. of ginger (minced)
- One-third tsp. of honey
- One-fourth cup of ice cubes
- One pinch of salt
- Two tsps. of vanilla extract
- Three-fourth cup of water
- One cup of zucchini (chopped)

Method:

1. Add all the listed ingredients in a high power blender. Blend for two minutes until creamy and smooth.

2. Pour the smoothie in serving glasses and serve.

Carrot Peach Smoothie

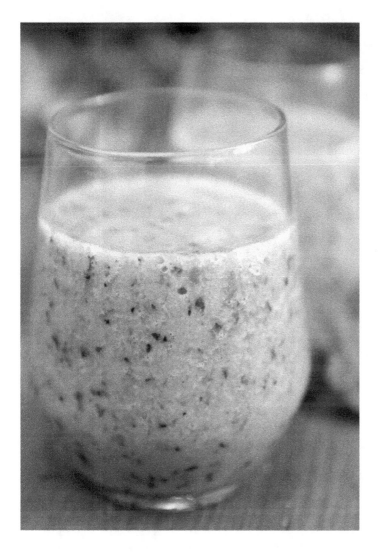

Total Prep & Cooking Time: Ten minutes

Yields: Two servings

Nutrition Facts: Calories: 191.2 | Protein: 11.2g | Carbs: 34.6g | Fat: 2.7g | Fiber: 5.4g

Ingredients

- Two cups of peach
- One cup of baby carrots
- One banana (frozen)
- Two tbsps. of Greek yogurt
- One and a half cup of coconut water
- One tbsp. of honey

Method:

1. Add peach, baby carrots, and banana in a high power blender. Blend on high settings for one minute.

2. Add Greek yogurt, honey, and coconut water. Give the mixture a whizz.

3. Pour the smoothie in glasses and serve.

Sweet Potato and Mango Smoothie
Total Prep & Cooking Time: Ten minutes

Yields: Two servings

Nutrition Facts: Calories: 133.3 | Protein: 3.6g | Carbs: 28.6g | Fat: 1.3g | Fiber: 6.2g

Ingredients

- One small sweet potato (cooked, smashed)
- Half cup of mango chunks (frozen)
- Two cups of coconut milk
- One tbsp. of chia seeds
- Two tsps. of maple syrup
- A handful of ice cubes

Method:

1. Add mango chunks and sweet potato in a high power blender. Blend until frothy and smooth.

2. Add chia seeds, coconut milk, ice cubes, and maple syrup. Blend again for one minute.

3. Divide the smoothie in glasses and serve.

Carrot Cake Smoothie

Total Prep & Cooking Time: Ten minutes

Yields: Two servings

Nutrition Facts: Calories: 289.3 | Protein: 3.6g | Carbs: 47.8g | Fat: 1.3g | Fiber: 0.6g

Ingredients

- One cup of carrots (chopped)
- One banana
- Half cup of almond milk
- One cup of Greek yogurt
- One tbsp. of maple syrup
- One tsp. of cinnamon (ground)
- One-fourth tsp. of nutmeg
- Half tsp. of ginger (ground)
- A handful of ice cubes

Method

1. Add banana, carrots, and almond milk in a blender. Blend until frothy and smooth.

2. Add yogurt, cinnamon, maple syrup, ginger, nutmeg, and ice cubes. Blend again for two minutes.

3. Divide the smoothie in serving glasses and serve.

Notes:

- You can add more ice cubes and turn the smoothie into slushy.

- You can store the leftover smoothie in the freezer for two days.

Chapter 4: Green Smoothies

Green smoothies can help in the process of detoxification as well as weight loss. Here are some easy-to-make green smoothie recipes for you.

Kale Avocado Smoothie

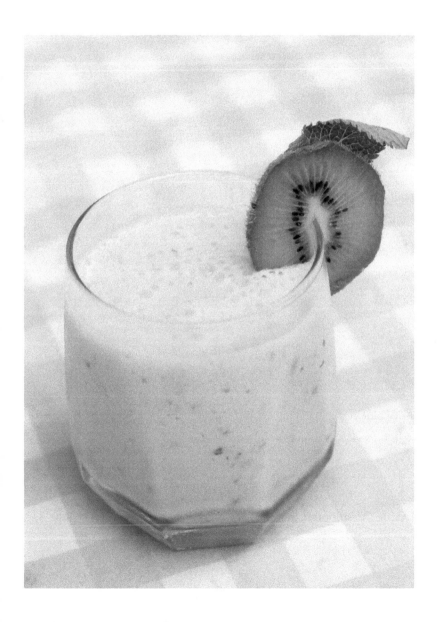

Total Prep & Cooking Time: Ten minutes

Yields: Two servings

Nutrition Facts: Calories: 401 | Protein: 11.2g | Carbs: 64.6g | Fat: 17.3g | Fiber: 10.2g

Ingredients

- One banana (cut in chunks)
- Half cup of blueberry yogurt
- One cup of kale (chopped)
- Half ripe avocado
- One-third cup of almond milk

Method:

1. Add blueberry, banana, avocado, and kale in a blender. Blend for making a smooth mixture.

2. Add the almond milk and blend again.

3. Divide the smoothie in glasses and serve.

Celery Pineapple Smoothie

Total Prep & Cooking Time: Ten minutes

Yields: Two servings

Nutrition Facts: Calories: 112 | Protein: 2.3g | Carbs: 3.6g | Fat: 1.2g | Fiber: 3.9g

Ingredients

- Three celery stalks (chopped)
- One cup of cubed pineapple
- One banana
- One pear
- Half cup of almond milk
- One tsp. of honey

Method:

1. Add celery stalks, pear, banana, and cubes of pineapple in a food processor. Blend until frothy and smooth.

2. Add honey and almond milk. Blend for two minutes.

3. Pour the smoothie in serving glasses and enjoy!

Cucumber Mango and Lime Smoothie

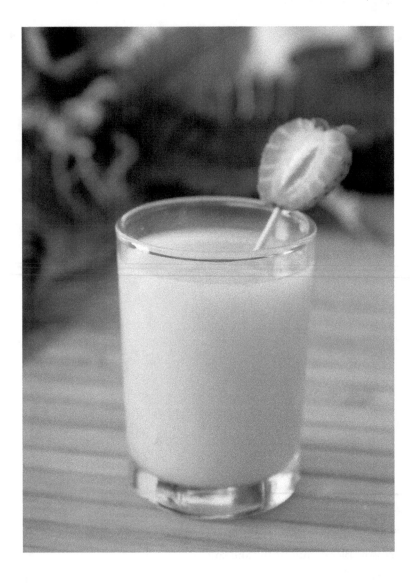

Total Prep & Cooking Time: Ten minutes

Yields: Two servings

Nutrition Facts: Calories: 165 | Protein: 2.2g | Carbs: 32.5g | Fat: 4.2g | Fiber: 3.7g

Ingredients

- One cup of ripe mango (frozen, cubed)
- Six cubes of ice
- Half cup of baby spinach leaves
- Two leaves of mint
- Two tsps. of lime juice
- Half cucumber (chopped)
- Three-fourth cup of coconut milk
- One-eighth tsp. of cayenne pepper

Method:

1. Add mango cubes, spinach leaves, and cucumber in a high power blender. Blend until frothy and smooth.

2. Add mint leaves, lime juice, coconut milk, cayenne pepper, and ice cubes. Process the ingredients until smooth.

3. Pour the smoothie in glasses and serve.

Kale, Melon, and Broccoli Smoothie

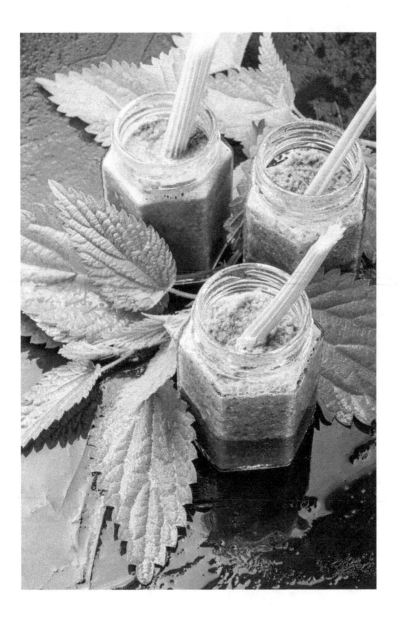

Total Prep & Cooking Time: Ten minutes

Yields: One serving

Nutrition Facts: Calories: 96.3 | Protein: 2.3g | Carbs: 24.3g | Fat: 1.2g | Fiber: 2.6g

Ingredients

- Eight ounces of honeydew melon
- One handful of kale
- Two ounces of broccoli florets
- One cup of coconut water
- Two sprigs of mint
- Two dates
- Half cup of lime juice
- Eight cubes of ice

Method:

1. Add kale, melon, and broccoli in a food processor. Whizz the ingredients for blending.

2. Add mint leaves and coconut water. Blend again.

3. Add lime juice, dates, and ice cubes. Blend the ingredients until smooth and creamy.

4. Pour the smoothie in a smoothie glass. Enjoy!

Kiwi Spinach Smoothie

Total Prep & Cooking Time: Ten minutes

Yields: Two servings

Nutrition Facts: Calories: 102 | Protein: 3.6g | Carbs: 21.3g | Fat: 2.2g | Fiber: 3.1g

Ingredients

- One kiwi (cut in chunks)
- One banana (cut in chunks)
- One cup of spinach leaves
- Three-fourth cup of almond milk
- One tbsp. of chia seeds
- Four cubes of ice

Method:

1. Add banana, kiwi, and spinach leaves in a blender. Blend the ingredients until smooth.

2. Add chia seeds, ice cubes, and almond milk. Blend again for one minute.

3. Pour the smoothie in serving glasses and serve.

Avocado Smoothie

Total Prep & Cooking Time: Ten minutes

Yields: Two servings

Nutrition Facts: Calories: 345 | Protein: 9.1g | Carbs: 47.8g | Fat: 16.9g | Fiber: 6.7g

Ingredients

- One ripe avocado (halved, pitted)
- One cup of milk
- Half cup of vanilla yogurt
- Eight cubes of ice
- Three tbsps. of honey

Method:

1. Add avocado, vanilla yogurt, and milk in a blender. Blend the ingredients until frothy and smooth.

2. Add honey and ice cubes. Blend the ingredients for making a smooth mixture.

3. Serve immediately.

PART II

Chapter 1: What Is Fasting?

Introduction to Fasting

Latest Research and Studies about Fasting

In a research published by the Springer Journal, it was found that fasting helps fight against obesity. The study, led by Kyoung Han Kim and Yun Hye Kim, was aimed at tracking the effects of fasting on fat cells. They put a group of mice into a four-month period of intermittent fasts, where the mice were fed for two days, followed by a day of fasting. In the end, the group of fasting mice was found to weigh less than the non-fasting mice, even though all of them had consumed exact quantities of food. The group of fasting mice had registered a drop in the fat buildup around fat cells. The explanation was that the fat had been converted into energy when glucose was insufficient. (www.sciencedaily.com/releases/2017/10/171017110041.htm)

In November 2017, Harvard researchers established that fasting can induce a long life, as well as minimize aging effects. It was found that fasting revitalizes mitochondria. Mitochondria are the organelles that act as body power plants. In this replenished state, mitochondria optimize physiological functions, in effect slowing down the aging process. Fasting also promotes low blood glucose levels, which improves skin clarity and boosts the immune system. (https://newatlas.com/fasting-increase-lifespan-mitochondria-harvard/52058/)

Sebastian Brandhorst, a researcher based at the University of Southern California, found out that fasting has a positive impact on brain health. Fasting induces low blood sugar levels, causing the liver to produce ketone bodies that pass on to the brain in place of sugars. Ketone bodies are much more stable and efficient energy sources than glucose. Researchers from the same university have posited that fasting minimizes chances of coming down with diabetes and other degenerative diseases. Moreover, they discovered that fasting induces low production of the IGF-1 hormone, which is a catalyst in aging and spread of disease. (https://www.cnbc.com/2017/10/20/science-diet-fasting-may-be-more-important-than-just-eating-less.html)

Biological Effects of Fasting

- **Cleanses the body**

Our bodies harbor an endless count of toxins, and these toxins announce their presence through symptoms like low energy, infections, allergies, terrible moods, bloating, confusion, and so on.

Eliminating toxins from your body will do you a world of good in the sense that your body will upgrade and start functioning optimally. There are many ways to cleanse your body: hydrotherapy, meditation, organic diets, herbs, yoga, etc.

But one of the most effective ways of cleansing your body is through fasting. When you go on a fast, you allow the body to channel the energy that would have been used for digestion into flushing out toxins.

- **Improves heart health**

Studies show that people who undertake regular fasts are less likely to contract coronary infections. Fasting fights against obesity, and obesity is a recipe for heart disease. It purifies the blood too, in that sense augmenting the flow of blood around the body.

- **Improves the immune system**

Fasting rids the body of toxins and radicals, thus boosting the body's immune system and minimizes the chances of coming down with degenerative diseases like cancer. Fasting reduces inflammation as well.

- **Improves bowel movement**

One of the problems of consuming food on the regular is that the food sort of clogs up your stomach, causing indigestion. You might go for days without visiting the bathroom to perform number two. But when you fast, your body resources won't be bogged down by loads of undigested foods, and so your bowel movement will be seamless. Also, fasting promotes healthy gut bacteria.

- **Induces alertness**

When your stomach is full because of combined undigested foods (i.e., "garbage"), you are more likely to experience brain-fog. You won't have any concentration on the tasks at hand. You will just sit around and laze the hours away, belching and spitting. But when you fast, your mind will be clear so it will be easy to cultivate focus.

Treating Fasting as a Lifestyle Choice

When you perform a simple Google search for the word "fasting," millions of results come up. Fasting is slowly becoming a mainstream subject. This is mostly because of the research-backed evidence that has been published by many reputable publications listing down the various benefits of fasting such as improved brain health, increased production of the human growth hormone, a stronger immune system, heart health, and weight loss—thus its appeal to health-conscious people as a catalyst for their health goals.

Taking up fasting as a lifestyle choice will see you go without food for anywhere from a couple of hours to days. But before you get into it, you'd do yourself a world of good to first obtain clearance from a physician, certifying that your body is ready, because not everyone is made for it. For instance, the symptoms of illnesses such as cancer may worsen after a long stretch of food deprivation. So people with degenerative diseases such as cancer should consider getting professional help or staying away altogether. Pregnant women, malnourished people, and children are advised to stay clear too.

The first thing you must do is to establish your fasting routine. For instance, you may choose to skip breakfast, making lunch your first meal of the day. Go at it with consistency. Also, you may decide to space your meals over some hours; so that when the set hours elapse, you reach your eating window, and then go back to fasting. The real challenge is staying committed. You will find that it will be difficult to break the cycle of eating that your body had been accustomed to, but when you persevere; your body will, of course, adjust to your new habit. If you decide to go for days without food, the results will be far pronounced, but please remember to hydrate your body constantly to flush out toxins.

Summary

Fasting is the willing abstinence from food over a period of time with the goal of improving your life. Conventionally, fasting has been tied to religious practices, but a new school of thought has emerged to proclaim the health benefits of fasting—particularly, weight loss. When you go into a fast, you create a caloric deficit, which triggers the body to convert its fat stores into energy. Numerous studies by mainstream health organizations have been done on fasting, and researchers have established that fasting has a host of advantages like improved motor skills, cognition, and moods. Some of the biological effects of fasting include improved bowel movement, immune system, and heart health. If you are starting out with fasting, you must create a routine and abide by it. Not everyone is fit to practice fasting. Some of the people advised to stay away from the practice include extremely sick people, pregnant women, the malnourished, and children. If you undertake a prolonged fast, you should hydrate your body constantly.

Chapter 2: Obesity and the Standard American Diet

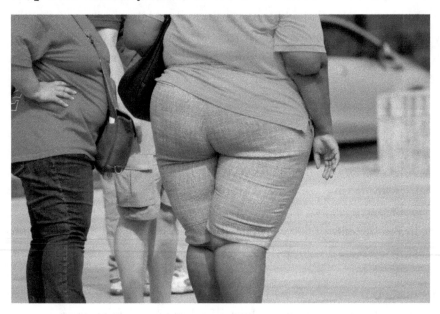

The Obesity Epidemic

We are killing ourselves with nothing more than a spoon and a fork. In 2017, obesity claimed more lives than car accidents, terrorism, and Alzheimer's combined. And the numbers are climbing at a jaw-dropping rate. Obesity has become a crisis that we cannot afford to ignore anymore.

You'd be mistaken to think that obesity is a crisis in first-world economies alone. Even developing nations are experiencing an upsurge of obese citizens. Here comes the big question: what is the **main** force behind this epidemic?

According to new research published in the New England Journal of Medicine, excessive caloric intake and lack of exercise are to blame.

Most American fast food chains have now become global. Fast foods, which are particularly calorie-laden, appeal to a lot of people across the world because of their low prices and taste. So, most people get hooked on the fast food diet and slowly begin the plunge into obesity.

The United States recognizes obesity as a health crisis and lawmakers have petitioned for tax increment on fast foods and sugary drinks, except that for a person who's addicted to fast foods, it would take a lot more than a price increase to discourage their food addiction. It would take a total lifestyle change.

Exercising alone won't help you; no matter how powerful your reps may be, or leg lifts or anything else you try in the gym, nothing can save you from a terrible diet.

And here's the complete shocker; the rate of childhood obesity has surpassed adulthood obesity; a terrible, terrible situation considering that childhood obesity almost always leads to heart complications in adult life.

Why Are We So Fat?

- **Poor food choices**

The number one reason why we are so fat is our poor choice of food. We eat too much of the wrong food, and most of it is not expended, so it becomes stored up as fat.

- **Bad genetics**

It's true that some people are genetically predisposed to gain more weight. Their genetics have wired them to convey abnormal hunger signals, so their bodies pressure them into consuming much more food.

- **Lack of strenuous activities**

Our modern-day lives involve only light physical tasks. Contrast that with the era of the dawn of humanity. Back then people would use up a lot of energy to perform physical activities and survive in unforgiving habitats.

Most of the food they consumed would be actually utilized. But today, thanks to our technological advancement, we have been spared from taking part in laborious activities. This makes it hard to use up the energy from food, and the body opts to store it as fat.

- **Psychological issues**

Some of us react to bad moods by indulging in food—in particular, high-calorie fast foods—because the taste of fast foods appeals to our unstable emotions. When we fall in the habit of rewarding our bad moods or depression with binge eating, we unsuspectingly fall into the trap of food addiction, to the point of getting depressed when we fail to binge eat, kicking off our journey into obesity.

- **The endocrine system**

The thyroid's hormones play a critical role in the metabolic rate of a person. Ideally, a strong endocrine system means a high metabolic rate. And so, individuals who have a weakened endocrine system are much more likely to develop obesity.

The Problem with Calories

Calories are the basic units for quantifying the energy in the food we consume. A healthy man needs a daily dose of around 2500 calories to function optimally, and a woman needs 2000 calories.

This caloric target should be met through the consumption of various foods containing minerals, vitamins, antioxidants, fiber, and other important elements, and this is not hard at all to achieve if you adhere to the old-fashioned "traditional diet."

But the challenge is that nowadays, we have many foods with a high caloric count, and yet they hardly fill us up! For instance, fries, milkshake, and a burger make up nearly 2000 calories! You can see how easy it'd be to surpass the caloric limit by indulging in fast food.

When we consume more calories than we burn, our bodies store up the excess calories as fat, and as this process repeats itself over time, the fat has a compounding effect that leads to weight gain.

The only way to make your weight stable is through balancing out the energy you consume with the energy you expend. But for someone who suffers from obesity, if they'd like to have a normal weight, they must create a caloric deficit, and fasting is the surefire practice of creating such a deficit.

Besides checking your caloric intake, you might also consider improving your endocrine system and the efficiency of both your kidney and liver, because they have a direct impact on how the body burns calories. When you buy food products, always find out their caloric count to assess how well they'll fit within your daily caloric needs.

The American Diet

In a 2016 lifestyle survey, most Americans admitted that it is not easy to keep their diet clean and healthy. This isn't surprising, especially when you consider the fact that the average American consumes more than 20 pounds of sweeteners each year. The over-emphasis of sugar and fat in the American diet is the leading cause of obesity in Americans. Illnesses triggered by obesity long started marching into our homes. What we have now is a crisis. But let's find out the exact types of foods that Americans like to feast on (we are big on consuming, it's no secret).

As a melting point of cultures drawn from various parts of the world, it's kind of difficult to say exactly what the all-American favorite foods are. But the United States Department of Agriculture might shine some light on this. It listed down desserts, bread, chicken, soda, and alcohol, as the top five sources of calories among Americans. As you can see, the sugar intake is impossibly high. Interestingly, the US Department of Agriculture also noted that Americans aren't big on fruits.

Pizza may qualify as the all-time favorite snack of America, followed closely by burgers and other fast food. There is a reason why most fast food restaurants are successful in America and throughout the world.

It has also been established that the average American drinks about a gallon of soda every week. Even drinks that are supposed to have a low-calorie count end up being calorie-bombs because of the doctoring that takes place. For instance, black coffee is low on calorie, but not so if it has milk and ice cream and sugar all over it.

Summary

The first-world economies are not alone in facing the crisis of obesity. It has emerged that people in poor countries are battling obesity too. Obesity-related deaths are on the rise. In 2017, the figures were especially shocking, for they'd surpassed the death count of terrorist attacks, accidents, and Alzheimer's combined. One of the corrective measures that the US government is considering to undertake is tax increment on sugars. The chief reason why we are so fat is our poor diets. Our foods are laden with sugars and fats, and it doesn't help that our lifestyles allow us to expend only a small amount of energy, which leads to fat accumulation and consequent weight gain. The average man requires around 2500 calories for his body to act optimally whereas the average woman requires 2000 calories. The top five daily sources of calories for Americans include desserts, bread, chicken, soda, and alcohol.

Chapter 3: Benefits of Fasting

Improved Insulin Sensitivity

Insulin sensitivity refers to how positively or negatively your body cells respond to insulin. If you have a high insulin sensitivity, you will need less amount of insulin to convert the sugars in your blood into energy, whereas someone with low insulin sensitivity would need a significantly larger amount of insulin.

Low insulin sensitivity is characterized by increased blood sugar levels. In other words, the insulin produced by the body is underutilized when converting sugars into energy. Low insulin sensitivity may make you vulnerable to ailments such as cancer, heart disease, type 2 diabetes, stroke, and dementia.

Ailments and bad moods are the general causes of low insulin sensitivity. However, high insulin sensitivity is restored once the ailments and bad moods are over.

Fasting is shown to have a positive effect on insulin sensitivity, enhancing your body to use small amounts of insulin to convert blood sugar into energy.

Improved insulin sensitivity has a great impact on health: leveling up physiological functions and fighting off common symptoms of ailments like lightheadedness and lethargy.

To increase insulin sensitivity, here are some of the best practices: perform physical activities, lose weight, consume foods that are high in fiber and low in Glycemic load, improve your moods and alleviate depressed feelings, and finally, make sure to improve the quality of your sleep.

The rate of insulin sensitivity is also heavily dependent on lifestyle changes. For instance, if you take up sports and exercise, insulin sensitivity goes up, but if you become lazy and inactive, it goes down.

- **Increased Leptin Sensitivity**

Leptin is the hormone that determines whether you're experiencing hunger or full. This hormone plays a critical role in weight loss and health management, and if your body grows insensitive to it, you become susceptible to some ailments. Understanding the role of leptin in your body is critical as it goes into helping you improve your health regimen.

Whenever this hormone is secreted by the fat cells, the brain takes notice, and it tries to determine whether you are in need of food or are actually full. Leptin needs to work as normally as possible else you will receive an inaccurate signal that will cause you to either overfeed or starve yourself.

Low leptin sensitivity induces obesity. This condition is normally witnessed in people with high levels of insulin. The excessive sugars in blood are carried off by insulin into fat cells, but when there is an insulin overload, a communication crash is triggered between fat cells and the brain. This condition induces low leptin sensitivity. When this happens, your brain is unable to tell the exact amount of leptin in your blood, and as such it misleads you. Low leptin sensitivity causes the brain to continue sending out the hunger signal even after you are full. This causes you to eat more than you should and, given time, leads to chronic weight gain.

Fasting has been shown to increase leptin sensitivity, a state that allows the brain to be precise in determining blood leptin quantities, and ensures that the accurate signal is transmitted to control your eating habits.

- **Normalized Ghrelin Levels**

Known as the "hunger hormone," ghrelin is instrumental in regulating both appetite and the rate of energy distribution into body cells.

Increased levels of ghrelin cause the brain to trigger hunger pangs and secrete gastric acids as the body anticipates you to consume food.

It is also important to note that both ghrelin and leptin receptors are located on the same group of brain cells, even though these hormones play contrasting roles, i.e., ghrelin being the hunger hormone, and leptin the satiety hormone.

The primary role of ghrelin is to increase appetite and see to it that the body has a larger fat reservoir. So, high ghrelin levels in your blood will result in you wanting to eat more food and, in some cases, particular foods like cake or fries or chocolate.

People who have low ghrelin levels will not eat enough amounts of food and are thus vulnerable to diseases caused by underfeeding. As a corrective measure, such people should receive shots of ghrelin to restore accurate hunger signals in their bodies.

Studies show that obese people suffer from a disconnection between their brains and ghrelin cells, so the blood ghrelin levels go through the roof, which makes these people be in a state of perpetual hunger. So, these obese people respond to their hunger pangs by indulging in their foods of choice, and thus the chronic weight gain becomes hard to manage.

It has been proven that fasting has a positive effect on ghrelin levels. Fasting streamlines the faulty communication between the brain receptors and ghrelin cells. When this is corrected, the brain starts to send out accurate hunger signals, discouraging you from eating more than you should.

- **Increased Lifespan And Slow Aging**

A study by Harvard researchers demonstrated that intermittent fasting led to an increased lifespan and the slowing down of the aging process. These findings were largely hinged on the cell-replenishing effects of fasting and flushing out of toxins.

The average person puts their digestive system under constant load because they're only a short moment away from their next meal. And given the fact that most foods are bacteria-laden, the immune system becomes strained with all the wars that it must be involved in. This makes the body cells prone to accelerated demise. But what happens when you go on a fast?

The energy that would have previously gone into digesting food is used to flush out toxins from the body instead. Also, it has been observed that body cells are strengthened during a fast, which makes physiological functions a bit more robust.

Fasting also enhances the creation of new neural pathways and regeneration of brain cells. This goes towards optimizing the functions of your brain. And, as we know, an energetic brain makes for a "youthful" life.

When you are on a fast, the blood sugar levels are generally down. The skin responds favorably to low blood sugar levels by improving elasticity and keeping wrinkles at bay. A high blood sugar level is notorious for making you ashy and wrinkly.

Fasting may increase your lifespan even from an indirect perspective. For instance, fasting may develop your sense of self-control, improve your discipline, and even increase your creativity. These immaterial resources are very necessary for surviving in the real world.

- **Improved Brain Function**

Fasting triggers the body to destroy its weak cells in a process known as autophagy. One of the main benefits of autophagy is reducing inflammation. Also, autophagy makes way for new and healthy body cells. Autophagy promotes neurogenesis, which is the creation of new brain cells.

Fasting allows the body to deplete the sugars in the blood, and since the body must continue to operate lest it shuts down, the body turns to an alternative energy source: fats. Through the aid of the liver, ketone bodies are produced to supply energy to the brain. Ketone bodies are a much cleaner and reliable source of energy than carbohydrates. Ketone bodies are known to tone down the effects of inflammatory diseases like arthritis.

Fasting promotes high insulin sensitivity. In this way, the body uses less insulin to convert sugars into energy. High insulin sensitivity means that the body will send out accurate signals when it comes to informing the host of either hunger or satiation.

Fasting enhances the production of BDNF (Brain-Derived Neurotrophic Factor), which a plays a critical part in improving neuroplasticity. And thus more resources are committed to the functions of the brain. BDNF is responsible for augmenting areas like memory, learning, and emotions.

Fasting supercharges your mind. It does so through facilitating the creation of new mitochondria. And since mitochondria are the power plants of our bodies, the energy output goes up. This increase in energy and resources causes the brain to function at a much higher level and yields perfect results.

- **Improved Strength And Agility**

When you think of a person that is considered strong and agile, your mind might conceive a well-muscled individual with veins bulging out their neck. Strength and agility come down to practice and more practice. The easiest way to develop agility and strength is obviously through physical training and sticking to a routine until your body adapts.

You must practice every day to be as strong and agile as you'd want to be. Also, you must take particular care over your dietary habits. Professional athletes stick to a diet that has been approved by their doctors for a reason. When it comes to developing strength and agility, nothing matches the combination of exercise and a flawless diet.

But besides fulfilling these two requirements, fasting, too, has its place. Did you know that you can amplify your strength and agility through fasting?

Fasting provokes the body to secrete the Human Growth Hormone. This hormone enhances organ development and even muscle growth. So when you fast, the HGH hormone might be secreted, and it will amplify the effects of your exercise and diet regimen, making you many times stronger and agile.

Fasting will promote the renewal of your body cells and thus lessen the effects of inflammation. When you perform physical exercises, you're basically injuring and damaging your body cells. So, when you fast, you'll allow your body to destroy its weak cells, and make room for new body cells through biogenesis.

Additionally, fasting will go a long way toward improving your motor skills, making you walk with the grace of a cat, with your body parts flexible.

- **Improved Immune System**

The immune system is responsible for defending your body against organisms that are disease vectors. When a foreign organism enters your body, and the body considers it harmful, the immune system immediately comes into action.

Some of the methods suggested for improving the immune system include having a balanced diet, quality sleep, improving your mental health, and taking physical exercises.

Fasting is an understated method of boosting your immune system.

In a research conducted by scientists at the University of Southern California, it emerged that fasting enhanced the rejuvenation of the immune system. Specifically, new white blood cells were formed, strengthening the body's defense system.

The regeneration of the immune system is especially beneficial to people who have a weak body defense mechanism—namely, the elderly, and the sick. This could probably be the reason why an animal in the wild responds to illness by abstaining from food.

In the same study, it was shown that there is a direct correlation between fasting and diminished radical elements in the body. Cell biogenesis was responsible for eradicating inflammation. And moreover, a replenished immune system discouraged the growth of cancer cells.

Depending on how long you observe a fast, the body will, at one point, run out of sugars, and then it will turn to your fat reservoirs to provide energy for its many physiological functions. Fats make for a much cleaner and stable and resourceful energy source than sugars ever will.

So, relying on this fat-energy, the immune system tends to function at a most optimal level.

- **Optimized Physiological Functions**

These are some of the body's physiological functions: sweating, bowel movement, temperature regulation, urinating, and stimuli response.

In a healthy person, all physiological functions should be seamless, but that cannot be said for most of us because our lifestyles get in the way.

So, the next time you rush to the bathroom intending to take a number two only to wind up spending half an hour there, you might want to take a close look at what you are eating.

Fasting is a great method of optimizing your physiological functions. When you observe a normal eating schedule, your body is under constant strain to keep digesting food—a resource-intensive process. But when you go on a fast, the energy that would have been used for digesting food will now be channeled into other critical functions. For instance, the body may now start ridding itself of radicals that promote indigestion, or amp up the blood circulation system, or even devote energy toward enhancing mental clarity, with the result being optimized physiological functions.

With more resources freed up from the strain of digestion, physiological processes will continue seamlessly, and once the glycogen in the blood is over, the body will continue to power physiological functions with energy acquired from fat cells.

The cellular repair benefits attached to fasting enables your body to perform its functions way better. Fasting reduces oxidative stress, which is a key accelerator of aging. In this way, fasting helps restore the youthfulness of your body cells, and the cells are very much optimized for performance.

- **Improved Cardiovascular Health**

When we talk about cardiovascular health, we are essentially talking about the state of the heart, and specifically, its performance in blood circulation.

Factors that improve the condition of your heart include a balanced diet, improved emotional and mental state, quality sleep, and living in a good environment. When cardiovascular health is compromised, it might lead to fatal consequences.

Researchers have long established that fasting improves cardiovascular health.

One of the outcomes of fasting is cholesterol reduction. The lesser cholesterol you have in your blood, the more seamless the movement of blood through your body. Complications are minimal or nonexistent. Thus your heart will be in a great condition.

Fasting also plays a critical role in toning down diabetes. The average diabetic tends to have low insulin sensitivity. For that reason, they need more insulin than is necessary to convert sugars into energy. It puts a strain on body organs and especially the pancreas. This might cause a trickle-down complication that goes back to the heart.

When the body enters fasting mode, it starts using up the stored energy to fulfill other important physiological functions such as blood circulation, in this way boosting the effectiveness of the heart.

Fasting helps you tap into your "higher state." The effects of matured spiritual energy and peaceful inner self cannot be gainsaid. Someone who's at peace with both himself and the universe is bound to develop a very healthy heart, as opposed to one who's constantly bitter, and one who feels as though he's drowning in a bottomless pit.

- **Low Blood Pressure**

People who have a high blood pressure are at risk of damaging not only their heart but their arteries too. When the pressure of the blood flowing in your arteries is high over a long period of time, it is bound to damage the cells of your arteries, and in the worst case scenario, it might trigger a rupture, and cause internal bleeding. High blood pressure puts you at risk of heart failure. Your heart might overwork itself and slowly start wearing out, eventually grinding to a halt.

In people with high blood pressure, a bigger-than-normal left heart is common, and the explanation is that their left heart struggles to maintain the cardiovascular output. So it starts bulking up and eventually creates a disrupting effect on your paired organ. Another risk associated with high blood pressure is coronary disease. This ailment causes your arteries to thin out to the point that it becomes a struggle for blood to flow into your heart. The dangers of coronary disease include arrhythmia, heart failure, and chest pain.

I started by mentioning the risks of high blood pressure because observing a fast normalizes your blood pressure. With a normal blood pressure, you can reverse these risks. Also, normal blood pressure improves the sensitivity of various hormones like ghrelin and leptin, eliminating the communication gap between brain receptors and body cells.

The low blood pressure induced by fasting causes you to have improved motor skills. It is common to hear people admit that fasting makes them feel light and flexible.

- **Decreased Inflammation**

Inflammation is an indication that the body is fighting against an infectious organism. It causes the affected parts to appear red and swollen.

Many diseases that plague us today are rooted in inflammation, and by the look of things, inflammation will be stuck with us for longer than we imagine.

The role of inflammation in mental health cannot be understated. Inflammation is to blame for bad moods, depression, and social anxiety.

The good news though is that fasting can reduce inflammation. Fasting has been shown to be effective in treating mental problems that are rooted in inflammation and as well as safeguarding neural pathways.

Individuals who have incorporated fasting into their lives are much less likely to suffer breakdowns and bad moods than people who don't fast at all.

Asthma, a lung infection, also has an inflammatory background. What's interesting is that fasting alleviates the symptoms of asthma.

The level of hormone sensitivity determines absorption rates of various elements into body cells. For instance, low insulin sensitivity worsens the rate of conversion of sugar into energy. Fasting improves insulin sensitivity, and thus more sugars can be converted into energy.

Fasting enhances the brain to form new pathways when new information is discovered. In this way, your memory power receives a boost, and you are better placed to handle stress and bad thoughts.

Fasting is very efficient in alleviating gut inflammation. Constant fasting promotes healthy gut flora which makes for great bowel movements.

Fasting is a great means of reducing heart inflammation, too. It does so through stabilizing blood pressure and fighting off radical elements.

- **Improved Skin Care**

Most of us are very self-conscious about how we look to the world. Bad skin, acne, and other skin ailments can be a real bother. Fasting has numerous benefits when it comes to improving your skin health, and it is said that fasting bestows a glow on your face. Experts claim that skin ailments develop as a result of terrible stomach environments and that there is a correlation between gut health and skin quality. Fasting promotes the development of gut flora. In this way, your gut health is improved, resulting in improved skin.

When you are on a fast and are taking water, you will eliminate toxins from your body. The condition of your skin improves because the skin cells are free of harmful substances. Many people who previously suffered from a bad skin condition and had tried almost every treatment with no success have admitted that fasting was the only thing that worked.

Another benefit of fasting is that it slows down the aging process. The water consumed during the fast goes to flush out toxins, consequently reducing the effects of old age on your skin. Fasting also promotes low blood sugar. Low blood sugar promotes optimized physiological processes and, as a result, toning down the effects of aging.

When you go on a fast, the body allocates energy to areas that might have previously been overlooked. So, your bad skin condition may be treated with the stored up energy, and considering that the energy produced from fat is more stable and resourceful; your skin health will improve.

- **Autophagy**

This is the process whereby the body rids itself of weakened and damaged cells. Autophagy is triggered by dry fasting. The body simply "eats" the weakened cells to provide water to the healthy cells. Eliminated cells are usually weak and damaged. And their absence creates room for new cells that are obviously going to be powerful.

Autophagy has been shown to have many benefits, and they include:

- **Slowing down aging effects**

The formation of wrinkles and body deterioration are some of the effects of aging. However, thanks to autophagy, these effects can be reversed, since the body will destroy its old and weakened cells and replace them with new cells.

- **Reducing inflammation**

Inflammation is responsible for many diseases affecting us today, but thanks to autophagy, the cells that have been affected by inflammation are consumed, giving room for new cells.

- **Conserving energy**

Autophagy elevates the body into a state of energy conservation. In this way, your body can utilize resources in a most careful manner.

- **Fighting infections**

The destruction of old and weak body cells creates room for fresh and powerful body cells. In that vein, old and weakened white blood cells are destroyed, and then new powerful white blood cells are formed. These new white new blood cells fortify the immune system.

- **Improving motor skills**

Autophagy plays a critical role in improving the motor skills of an individual. This goes toward boosting the strength and agility of a person. Energy drawn from the weak and damaged cells is way more resourceful than the energy drawn from sugars.

Summary

There are numerous benefits attached to fasting. One of them is increased insulin sensitivity. When the insulin sensitivity goes up, insulin resistance drops, and the body is now able to use less insulin to convert sugars into energy. Another benefit of fasting is improved leptin sensitivity. The leptin hormone is known as the satiation hormone, and it is responsible for alerting you when you are full. An improved ghrelin level is another benefit of fasting. The ghrelin hormone is known as the hunger hormone. It induces hunger pangs so that you may feed. Fasting lengthens your existence. This is largely because of neuroregeneration of cells and flushing out toxins. Fasting improves brain function, strengthens your body and boosts agility, strengthens your immune system, optimizes your physiological functions, improves cardiovascular health, lowers blood pressure, reduces inflammation, improves your skin, and promotes autophagy. As researchers carry out new experiments, more benefits of fasting are being uncovered.

Chapter 4: Myths and Dangers of Fasting

Fasting has gained widespread acceptance across the world. More people who are seeking to improve their health through alternative means are turning to fasting. As you might expect, the field has been marred with conspiracies, lies, half-truths, and outright ignorance. Some of the long-held myths and misconceptions about fasting include:

Fasting makes you overeat. This myth hinges on the idea that after observing a fast, an individual is bound to be so hungry that they will consume more food to compensate for the period they'd abstained from food.

The brain requires a steady supply of sugars. Some people say that the brain cannot operate normally in the absence of sugars. These people believe that the brain uses sugars alone to power its activities and any other source of energy would not be compatible. So when you fast, you'd be risking shutting down your brain functions.

Skipping breakfast will make you fat. Some people seem to treat breakfast as though it were an unexplained mystery of the Earth. They say breakfast is special. Anyone who misses breakfast cannot possibly have a healthy life. They say that if you skip breakfast, you will be under a heavy spell of cravings, and finally give in to unhealthy foods.

Fasting promotes eating disorders. Some people seem to think that fasting is the stepping stone for disorders like bulimia and anorexia. They complain that once you see the effects of fasting, you might want to "amplify" the effects which might make you susceptible to an eating disorder like anorexia.

Fasting will make you overeat. This is partly true. However, it is important to note that most people fall into the temptation of overeating because of their lack of discipline and not necessarily because of unrealistic demands of fasting. If you're fasting the proper way, no temptation is big enough to lead you astray, and after all, the temptation exists to test whether you're really disciplined.

The brain requires a steady supply of sugars. This myth perpetuates the notion that we should consume carbohydrates every now and again to keep the brain in working condition. Also, this myth suggests that the brain can only use energy derived from sugars and not energy derived from fats. When you go on a fast, and your body uses up all the glycogen, your liver produces ketone bodies that are passed on to your brain to act as an energy source.

Skipping breakfast will make you fat. There is nothing special about breakfast. You can decide to skip breakfast and adhere to your schedule and be able to get desired results. It's true that skipping breakfast will cause you to be tempted by cravings, but you're not supposed to give in, and in that case, you become the problem. Skipping breakfast will not make you fat. What will make you fat is you pouring more calories into your body than you will spend.

Fasting promotes eating disorders. If you have a goal in mind, you are supposed to stay focused on that goal. The idea that an individual would plunge into the world of eating disorders simply because they want to amplify the results of fasting sounds like weakness on the part of the individual and not a fault of the practice itself.

Dangers of Fasting

Just as with most things in life, there's both a positive and negative side to fasting. Most of these problems are amplified in people who either fast in the wrong way or people who clearly shouldn't be fasting.

So let's explore some of the risks that are attached to fasting.

- **Dehydration**

Chances are, you will suffer dehydration while observing a fast, and drinking regular cups of water won't make the situation any better. Well, this is because most of your water intake comes from the foods that you consume daily. When dehydration kicks in, you are bound to experience nausea, headaches, constipation, and dizziness.

- **Orthostatic Hypotension**

This is common in people who drink water during their fasts. Orthostatic Hypotension causes your body to react unfavorably when you move around. For instance, when you stand on your feet and walk around, you might experience dizziness and feel as though you're at the verge of blowing up into smithereens. Other symptoms include temporary mental blindness, lightheadedness, and vision problems. These symptoms make it hard for you to function in activities that demand precision and focus, e.g., driving.

- **Worsened medical conditions**

People who fast while they are sick put themselves at risk of worsening their condition. The fast may amplify the symptoms of their diseases. People with the following ailments should first seek doctor's approval before getting into fasting: gout, type 2 diabetes, chronic kidney disease, eating disorders, and heartburn.

- **Increased stress**

The habit of skipping meals might lead to increased stress. The body might respond to hunger by increasing the hormone cortisol which is responsible for high-stress levels. And when you are in a stressed mental state, it becomes difficult to function in your day to day life.

Summary

Although fasting has a lot of benefits, there is a dark side to it too, but the negative effects can be minimized or eliminated altogether when a professional is involved. Dehydration is one of the negative effects. Besides providing nutrients to the body, food is also an important source of water. So when you fail to correct this gap by drinking a lot more water, your body will fall into a state of dehydration. Orthostatic hypotension is another danger. This illness makes you feel dizzy and lightheaded, and so it makes it difficult for you to function in an activity that demands your focus and stamina. Fasting may amplify the symptoms of your disease depending on your age and the stage of your disease. For instance, people who suffer from illnesses like gout, diabetes, eating disorders, and heartburn should first seek the doctor's approval before going on a fast. Moreover, fasting may lead to an increase in stress levels.

Chapter 5: Safety, Side Effects, and Warning

The Safest and Enlightened Way of Fasting

As the subject of fasting becomes popular, more people are stating their opinions on it, and as you might expect, some people are for it, and others are against it.

The best approach toward fasting is not set in stone, but it is rather determined by factors such as your age and health status.

Before you get into fasting, there are some critical balances you need to consider first. One of them is your experience. If you have never attempted a fast before, then it is a bad idea to go straight into a 48-hour fast, because you are likely to water down the effects. As a beginner, you must always start with lighter fasts and build your way up into extended fasts. You could begin by skipping one meal, then two meals, and finally the whole day.

Another important metric when it comes to determining the appropriate space between your eating windows is your health status. For instance, you cannot be a sufferer of late-stage malaria and yet go on a fast, because it might create a multiplying effect on your symptoms. People who are malnourished or have eating disorders might want to find other ways of improving their health apart from fasting.

An essential thing to note is that we are not all alike. My body's response to a fast is not going to be the exact response of yours. Knowing this, always listen to your body. Sometimes, a water-fast might trigger a throat infection and make your throat swollen. In such a situation, it would be prudent to suspend the fast and take care of your throat, as opposed to sticking to your guns.

Side Effects of Fasting

Fasting might upset the physiological functions of a body. This explains the side effects that crop up when you go on a fast. It is also important to note that most of these side effects subside as your body grows accustomed to the fast.

- **Cravings**

Top on the list is cravings. When you go on a fast, the immediate response by the body is to elevate the "hunger hormone" and so, you will start craving for sweet unhealthy foods. If you are not the disciplined type, this is a huge pitfall that could negate the effects of your fast.

- **Headaches**

Headaches, too, are a side effect of fasting. Most people who are new to fasting are bound to experience a headache. One of the explanations for headaches is that it is the brain's response to a shift from relying on carbohydrates to ketone bodies as the alternative energy source. Regular consumption of water might mitigate the headache or eliminate it altogether.

- **Low energy**

Another side effect is low energy. When you fast, the body might interpret it as starving, and its first response will be conserving energy. So, there will be less energy for physiological functions. In this way, you will start feeling less energetic than before.

- **Irritability**

Irritability is also a side effect. Studies show that people who are new to fasting are bound to have foul moods as their body increases stress hormones and hunger hormones. However, if they can persist, the irritability will eventually go away, and make room for a happy mood as the body switches to its fat stores for energy.

Types of People That Should Not Fast

The ideal person to go on a fast is a healthy person. People with certain medical conditions may still go on a fast, but it is always prudent to seek the guidance of a medical professional. We have previously stated that fasting strengthens the immune system. So is it contradicting to discourage fasting when one is sick? No! You may fast but preferably under the instruction and supervision of a medical professional. However, there are cases when it is inappropriate to fast.

Infants and children. Putting kids on a fast is just wrong. Their bodies are not fully developed yet to withstand periods of hunger. Fasting would do them more damage than good. For instance, it might mess with their metabolism and have a negative impact on their growth curve.

Hypoglycemics. People with hypoglycemia have extremely low levels of blood sugar. Their bodies need a constant stream of sugars to sustain normal functions lest severe illnesses take reign. For that reason, hypoglycemics should not fast.

Pregnant and nursing women. These women need a lot of energy because their young ones are dependent on them. So, pregnant women and nursing women are encouraged to keep their blood sugar steady.

The malnourished. People who are underweight and malnourished should stay away from fasting. To start with, their bodies don't have sufficient fat. So, when they go on a fast, their body will destroy its cells in search of nutrients. Over time, the results could be fatal.

People with heartburn. People who experience severe heartburn should not fast. This is because heartburn is a very distressing thing and there is no guarantee it will subside even when your body adapts to fasting. So, it is better to stay clear.

Impaired immune system. Fasting may have the ability to renew the strength and utility of your immune system. But when we are talking about an impaired immune system where most of the white blood cells are hanging on a thin blade, then fasting cannot be of help. Such a person would be better off sticking to a healthy diet.

Other classes of people that shouldn't fast include those recovering from surgeries, people with eating disorders, depressed souls, and people with extreme heart disease.

Summary

For purposes of safety, always ensure that your body is prepared to withstand the effects of fasting. You may prepare by evaluating your health status, experience, and developing a great sense of self-awareness. Fasting may have its numerous benefits, but there is also a negative side to it because fasting comes with unpleasant side effects. The good thing though is that most of these side effects tend to subside once the body grows accustomed to your fasting routine. One of the side effects of fasting is getting a headache. A headache is triggered by the brain's adjustment from relying on carbohydrates as an energy source and switching to ketone bodies. It may be mitigated through constant consumption of water. Another side effect is cravings. Your body makes you want to eat fast foods very badly. Fasting may also make you irritable, but it is for only a short time and then a happy mood sets in. Fasting also makes you feel less energetic, which can be uninspiring. These are some of the people that shouldn't fast: hypoglycemics, infants, children, pregnant women, nursing women, the malnourished, people with extreme ailments, and those recovering from surgeries.

Part 2: Types of Fasting and How to Fast

Chapter 6: Intermittent Fasting

What Is Intermittent Fasting?

Nowadays, intermittent fasting is one of the most talked about practices in health improvement domains. Basically, intermittent fasting is about creating a routine where you eat only after a set period of time. Intermittent fasting has been shown to have numerous benefits such as improving motor skills, developing willpower, and brain functions. Most people are turning to the practice to achieve their health goals— specifically, weight loss.

The most common way of performing an intermittent fast is by skipping meals. In the beginning, you may decide to skip one of the main meals, and when your body adapts to two meals a day, you may then elevate to just one meal per day. During the fast, you are not supposed to partake of any food, but it is okay to drink water and other low-calorie drinks like black coffee or black tea.

Intermittent fasting allows you to indulge in the foods of your choice, but there's emphasis on avoiding foods that are traditionally bad for your health. The main thing is to give your body time to process food between your eating windows.

Polls answered by people who have adopted this lifestyle indicate that most of them are happy with the results. Intermittent fasting is a very effective means of weight loss as it improves the metabolic rate of the body, as well as triggers cell autophagy. The good thing about intermittent fasting is that it allows you to partake of your favorite foods without making you feel guilty, which is a contrast to fad diets that insist on eating things like raw food and plant-based foods.

How to Practice Intermittent Fasting

There are a couple of ways to practice intermittent fasting. These are the three most popular ways:

- **The 16/8 method**

In this method, you are supposed to fast for 16 hours. Your eating window is restricted to eight hours every day. For instance, you might choose to only eat between twelve noon and eight in the evening.

- **Eat-Stop-Eat**

This fast involves irregular abstinence from food for a full 24 hours. You might decide to practice this once or twice every week. But when you fast, you must wait for 24 hours to pass before you indulge in the next meal. The eat-stop-eat method is very effective in not only weight loss but also in flushing out toxins from the body over the 24 hours you abstained from food.

- **The 5:2 Diet**

This type of intermittent fasting demands that you devote two days every week where you'll consume not more than 600 calories. Considering that the daily caloric requirement for the average person is 2000–2500, this type of fast will create a caloric deficit, and there's going to be weight loss as the body taps into its fat reservoirs for energy.

- **Alternate-Day Fasting**

This type of fasting requires that you skip one day and fast the next day. Depending on the intensity you want, you might choose to have a zero calorie intake or restrict your calorie intake to not more than 600. Alternate-day fasting is suitable for people who have experience with fasting and only want to escalate to amplify the benefits. A newbie should start with small fasts.

Pros and Cons of Intermittent Fasting

Intermittent fasting helps you save up on weekly food costs. That's a big advantage in these hard economic times. Food can be a very expensive affair especially if you eat out.

Intermittent fasting allows you to focus on your life goals. The energy that would have gone into looking for or preparing your next meal is used up to attain your important goals. Intermittent fasting has the potential to improve your emotional being and reduce anxiety—all of which make your life more stress-free.

Intermittent fasting is doable and safe. This means that it is free of complications and there's nothing to hold back anyone that wants to go into it. This is unlike other methods of weight loss like fad diets where some foods might be hard to access or expensive, or you dislike them.

Intermittent fasting improves the body's sensitivity to insulin, and by extension, it improves the metabolic rate of your body.

Moving on to the cons—the biggest disadvantage of intermittent fasting is the social dynamics. For instance, you might be out with friends when they decide to "pop in a joint" and then it's going to be strange to explain that you won't eat or maybe you'll defy your fasting routine and eat anyway, in which case you have cheated yourself.

Intermittent fasting doesn't seem to have a coherent and stable method. There are so many variations that dilute the philosophy of fasting. It almost feels like I can even come out with my style and popularize it. So, intermittent fasting lacks in originality.

Finding Your Ideal Intermittent Fasting Plan

The first and most important thing is to determine your health condition. If your body can permit you to indulge in intermittent fasting then, by all means, go ahead. If you are a beginner, you should start small, which means don't go from regular meals and start practicing 24-hour fasts.

That's counterproductive. Make sure you have some experience before you fast for an extended period of time.

You'll find that what works for someone won't necessarily work for everybody else. So what's one supposed to do? Test, test, test. At one point you will find a variation of the intermittent fast that will fit perfectly into your life. It's all about finding what really works for you and then committing to the routine.

In my experience, I have found the 16:8 to be the best. This type of intermittent fast requires that you abstain from food for 16 hours and then indulge for 8 hours. For most followers of this routine, they like to have their eating window between 12:00 PM and 20:00 PM. The 16-hour fast will be inclusive of sleep, which makes it less severe.

This method is extremely efficient in weight loss, and most people have reported success. However, you must stick to the routine for a while before you can see any results. Don't do it for just one day and climb on the weighing machine only to find that there are no changes and then give up.

To improve the success of fasting intermittently, stick to a balanced diet during your eating windows, and don't take the fast as an excuse for indulging in unhealthy foods.

Step-By-Step Process of Fasting For a Week

The first step is to certify that you are in perfect condition. Get an appointment with your doctor and perform a whole health analysis to get a clean bill of health. Remember to always start with a small fast and gradually build up.

- **Day one**

When you wake up, forgo breakfast and opt for a glass of water or black coffee. Then go on about your work as you normally do. Around noon, your eating window opens. Now you are free to indulge in the food of your choice, but make sure that they are nutritious foods because unhealthy foods will water down your efforts. Your eating window should close at 20:00 PM, and from 20:01 pm to 12:00 pm the next day, don't consume anything else besides water.

- **Day two**

On day two, your body should have started to protest over the sudden calorie reduction, and so you'll be likely experiencing an irritable mood, lightheadedness, and a small headache. When you wake up, no matter how strong the urge to eat might be, just push it back, and the only thing you should consume is water or black coffee. At noon, your eating window opens, and you're free to eat until 8 pm.

- **Day three**

When you wake up, take a glass of water or black coffee. Chances are that your body has started to adjust to the reduced daily caloric intake. It has switched to burning fats. At twelve noon, when your eating window opens, consume less food than you did yesterday and the day before, so that the body has even lesser calories to work with. The body should adapt to this pretty swiftly.

- **Day four**

In the morning, take a glass of water or black coffee and go about your business. When your eating window opens, eat as much food as you ate yesterday, but in the evening, resist the urge to drink anything.

- **Day five**

When you wake up, take a glass of water or black coffee. During your eating window, eat less food than you did previously. At night, resist the urge to drink water.

- **Day six**

When you wake up, resist the urge to drink water or even coffee. In your eating window, choose not to eat at all, and at night give in to the temptation and drink water or black coffee.

- **Day seven**

When you wake up, take a glass of water or black coffee. In your eating window, resume eating, but only take a small portion, and just before you close the eating window, eat again, except it should be a slightly larger meal than previously. Before you sleep, take another glass of water or black coffee. Fast till your next eating window, and then you may resume your normal eating habits. At this point, you will have lost weight and experienced a host of other benefits attached to intermittent fasting.

Summary

Intermittent fasting features a cycle of fasting interrupted by an eating window. Some of the methods of intermittent fasting include the 16:8, eat-stop-eat, 5:2, and alternate-day fasting. The best approach to intermittent fasting is context-based in the sense that only you can know what works for you. The most popular form of intermittent fasting is the 16:8. In this method, you fast for 16 hours and then an eating window of 8 hours. The biggest advantage of intermittent fasting is that it announces relief to your pocket. The "food budget" goes into other uses. The amount of time that it takes to prepare meals is a real hassle, but intermittent fasting frees up your time so you can be more productive. The entry barrier is nonexistent too. This means anyone can practice intermittent fasting because there are no barriers or things to buy—a stark contrast to other weight loss methods like fad diets that may be both inconveniencing and expensive.

Chapter 7: Longer Periods of Fasting

What is Fasting for Longer Periods?

Fasting for longer periods is reserved for people who have a bit of experience with fasting. A newbie shouldn't get into it.

It is basically desisting from food for not less than 24 hours, but not more than, say, 48 hours. You may increase the success of the fast by making it a dry fast. In a dry fast, you won't have the luxury of drinking water or any other low-calorie drink like black coffee.

Fasting for longer periods requires that you prepare emotionally, mentally, and physically. The buildup to your fast is an especially important part. Your food consumption should be minimal.

Fasting for a longer period helps you achieve much more results because the body will be subjected to an increased level of strain.

However, you must take care to know when to stop. In some instances, the body might rebel by either catching an infection or shutting down critical functions, and in such times it is prudent to call off the fast.

During longer fasts, you should abstain from strenuous exercises, because the body will be in a state of energy conservation, and the available energy is purposed for physiological functions.

With the wrong approach, long fasts might become disastrous. That's why it is always important to seek clearance from your doctor first before you go into the fast. And to flush out toxins, ensure you have a steady intake of water.

It is estimated that weight loss in longer fasts averages around one to two pounds every day.

How to Fast for Longer Periods

The main reason that people go into longer fasts is to obviously lose weight. But you might want to fast to reach other purposes such as flushing toxins from your body or heightening your mental capabilities. Also, a longer fast is recommended if you are going into a surgery.

The response to a fast is different for everyone. If it is your first time, please take great care by getting medical clearance.

As your fast approaches, you might want to minimize your food consumption to get used to managing hunger.

Next, you should clear away items that might ruin your focus or tempt you to backslide. You might want to give your kitchen a total makeover by, for instance, clearing away the bad food. It is much easier to manage cravings when they are out of sight than when they are within easy reach.

Always start small. Before you deprive yourself food for over 24 hours, you should first get a taste of what food deprivation for 8 hours feels like, and if you can handle that, then you're ready to step up your game. While you fast, you should be very aware of the ranges of effects that your body experiences. You might feel dizzy, lightheaded, sleepy, or distressed, and these are okay reactions. Things that are not okay are infections and prolonged aches of body parts. If your body responds to fasting unfavorably, you should stop the fast.

Pros and Cons of Fasting for Longer Periods

If you have always been motivated to clear away the stubborn fat in your body, but have never found an efficient method, then the answer is to fast for a longer period.

When you go on a longer fast, the body uses up all glycogen in the first 24 hours, and then it switches to burning fats. A longer fast guarantees quick weight loss.

A longer fast saves you money. Food is an expensive affair, especially if you eat out. With a longer fast, it means you are staying away from food, and are thus saving on food costs.

Besides the benefit of optimizing your health, a longer fast will strengthen both your willpower and mental sharpness, which are two necessary factors in attaining success.

Fasting for a longer period helps you appreciate the taste of food. By the time you're done fasting, you'll want to indulge your appetite, and food will suddenly taste so sweet. The scarcity factor elevates the value of food.

A longer fast has cons, too. One of the biggest cons is the strain that it puts on your body. When your body goes from relying on glycogen into fats as a source of energy, nasty side effects are bound to come up—for instance, headaches, nausea, and lightheadedness.

Another con is that fasting for a longer period might open you up to disease. As much as fasting renews your immune system, your body still needs robust energy to function optimally. Fasting puts your body into a state of conserving energy which makes it easy for disease to attack.

Step-By-Step Process of Fasting for Longer Periods

When you decide to go on a fast for a longer period, you must realize that you are signing up for a real challenge. The body's immediate response to a fast is raising the hunger hormone to alert you to look for food. Now, fighting off that urge takes a lot of willpower. In some regard, it's why fasting might be considered a test of discipline because not so many people can withstand it.

So here's the step-by-step process of going on a fast for longer periods:

Preparation

The first major thing is to ensure that your body is in a condition that will allow you to fast, without any complications. In other words, consult your doctor for a checkup.

Reduce your food intake in the days leading up to your fast so that your body can get accustomed to staying without food. Once your body is familiar with the feeling of food deprivation, you are ready to move forward.

In the morning of your fast, drink lots of water. It is critical for flushing out toxins and reducing stomach acidity when your stomach secretes acids in anticipation of food. Your water intake should be regular and spread out through the day.

Rather than lying down and wearing a look of self-pity, just go on about your work as you normally would, provided it is not a very focus-oriented job like performing surgeries.

You should stay the whole day without food and then go to bed. On the following morning, your hunger pangs will be even more amplified, at which point you are to mitigate the hunger with a drink of water and then maintain the fast for another 24 hours. 48 hours are enough for a longer fast, and the weight loss should be dramatic. After the fast, don't immediately go back to eating heavy amounts of food, but rather ease your way into a lighter diet.

Chapter 8: Extended Fasting

How to Fast for Extended Periods

Fasting for an extended period is an extreme form of fasting that demands you abstain from food from anywhere between three days to seven days. If you can deny yourself food for more than three days, you should be proud of yourself, because not so many people have that kind of determination.

Fasting for an extended period of time amplifies the results of a longer fast. When you go for an extended period of time without food, you will allow yourself to experience a range of different feelings. At the initial stage there is distress, and towards the end your feelings become tranquil.

Considering that this is an especially long fast, you are supposed to take a very keen listen to the response by your body. If your body sends out the message that it is under massive strain, now it's time to stop the fast. Cases where it's appropriate to stop include developing stomach ulcers, throat infection, and loss of consciousness.

You should eat lighter meals as you approach the start of your fast. During the fast, your water intake should be regular. When you complete the fast, the transition to your normal eating life should be slow and gradual, starting with lighter meals.

Fasting for an extended period has the biggest potential of going wrong. The prolonged food deprivation in itself may do more good than harm. There is also the possibility of slightly altering your body's physiological functions. Still, the benefits of an extended fast outweigh the negatives.

Pros and Cons of Fasting for Extended Periods

The biggest advantage of fasting for an extended period of time is the discipline it instills in you. When you go for a prolonged period without eating food, your body will respond by increasing hunger pangs. It takes extreme willpower to keep going. This experience can help you build your self-control and discipline in real life.

An extended fast is very effective in banishing stubborn fat. Most people who are obese will tell you that they are trying to lose weight, but the fat is stubborn. Guess what, their methods are ineffective. However, if they had the will and courage to go on an extended fast, then they'd experience a rapid weight loss and reach their desired weight.

Extended fasting promotes a high rate of cell replenishing. When the body goes for days without food, it turns in on itself and begins to digest its cells—the weak and damaged cells—to provide nutrition for the healthy cells. The elimination of weak and damaged cells creates room for new and healthy ones.

The biggest disadvantage for an extended period of fasting is the risk of complications that you put your body into. Some complications might be instant whereas others may develop long after the fast. The biggest risk is catching an infection. If you're unlucky enough that you catch some disease in your fast, your immune system will be overwhelmed.

Another huge miss about extended fasting is the disconnect it encourages in your normal life. When you are fasting, you won't be able to share a meal with your friends or family, and that can be a big inconvenience. It can make people "talk."

Step-By-Step Process of Fasting for Extended Periods

When you get clearance from a medical professional, you should start by preparing for the extended fast. Ideally, if you are getting into an extended fast, you should have experience with either intermittent fasting, longer fasting or both. The more your body is familiar with food deprivation, the better the outcome.

On the start of your extended fast, you should consume only water or black coffee, and throughout the rest of the day, observe regular water consumption. It will aid in flushing out toxins and other harmful elements from your body.

During the fast, you should keep your normal work schedule, as opposed to being inactive, because inactivity will worsen your hunger pangs. The standard response to hunger pangs should be water consumption.

On the second day, first thing in the morning is to consume more water. This water is very critical in flushing out toxins and keeping your body cells hydrated as well as regulating autophagy. However, if you want to increase the success rate of the fast, you might consider eliminating water. One of the side effects of this type of fast is a dry mouth. A dry mouth has the potential of being very distressing. For purposes of safety, always hydrate yourself.

On the third day, wake up and consume water or black coffee. At this point, your body is subsisting on its fat reserves, and the weight loss is evident. Your body has potentially minimized hunger pangs to manageable levels. Keep yourself busy. Otherwise, inactivity will provoke hunger.

From the fourth day up until the seventh, keep the same routine. When you come to the end of your fast, realize that your body will be in starvation mode, so don't immediately consume large amounts of food. Instead, ease your way back into a normal eating schedule.

Chapter 9: The Eating Window

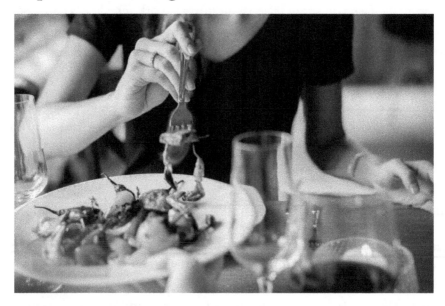

What is the Eating Window?

The eating window is the period of time that you are allowed to indulge in foods and one that precedes a period of fasting. The eating window comes around on a cycle, and you should adhere to it by only eating when the window opens and abstaining from food the rest of the time.

The hours are not set in stone. You are free to choose your eating window in a way that works for you. Most people who practice intermittent fasting seem to adhere to an eight-hour eating window followed by a sixteen-hour fast. Commonly, the eight-hour window opens at around 12:00 PM and goes all the way to 20:00 PM. During this time, you may indulge in your favorite foods. However, past 20:00 PM, you are supposed to observe the fast.

The 16:8 method of intermittent fasting appeals to many people because the 16 hours of fasting are inclusive of the bed-time. If you are not into waiting for sixteen hours before you partake of food, you may lessen the hours, so that you will have frequent eating windows between your fasts.

It is generally more fruitful to have a small eating window followed by a long period of fast.

It's also important to choose an eating window that optimizes your health. For instance, eating during the day is of much benefit than eating at night. This is because the body puts more calories to use during the day as opposed to while you are asleep. Also, adhere to a good diet, or else your gains will be neutralized by a bad diet.

What to Eat

The reason why intermittent fasting appeals to so many people is the nonexistent dietary rules common in alternative weight loss methods like fad diets. In intermittent fasting, you are free to eat the foods of your choice, and the main thing is to restrict your caloric intake.

You are free to consume the foods that delight you, but be careful not to fall in the pit of overcompensation. You are at risk of misleading yourself into consuming unhealthy foods during your eating window under the delusion that fasting will take care of it. Truth is, some of the fast foods we indulge are so calorie-laden that it would take a prolonged fast (not intermittent) to eliminate their fat from our bodies.

Limit your intake of red meat. As much as intermittent fasting is lenient when it comes to diet, it is widely known that red meat causes more harm than good. So, you might want to limit its intake or eliminate it altogether.

Fruits are a source of essential nutrients for the body. Always make sure to include fruits like bananas, avocados, and apples into your meals. Fruits help reduce inflammation and are critical in optimizing the physiological functions of the body.

Vegetables should be in your meals. People who claim that vegetables taste bad are just unimaginative cooks. Vegetables do taste good. And some of the health benefits of vegetable include strengthening your bones, stabilizing your blood sugar, boosting your brain health, and improving your digestive system.

Developing Discipline

It takes a lot of discipline to persevere through a fast. Think about it. The average person is accustomed to eating something every now and then. They cannot afford to hold back for even a couple more hours when lunch is due. The eating cycle never ends. And so a person who can decide to abstain from food and stick to their decision is a special kind of person—he/she is disciplined.

The biggest challenge when it comes to fasting for an extended period is to overcome the hunger pangs over the first few days. Your body floods you with the hunger hormone, pushing you to look for food. However, if you persevere through the first few days, your body will adjust to the food deprivation and switch to your stored fats as the alternative source of energy.

One of the things you must do to boost your self-control is to prepare your mind. When you have an idea of what to expect, the hunger will be more tolerable as opposed to if you're ignorant. Another thing to take into consideration is the weather. You don't want to fast during a cold season because fasting lowers your body temperature, and so you'll be hard-hit.

Another way of boosting your discipline is joining hands with people of the same goal. In this way, you can keep each other in check. When you are on a team or have a friend who practices fasting too, it will be easy to stick to your plan, as everybody will offer psycho-social support to everybody else. Sometimes, the difference between throwing in the towel and sticking to your guns is a kind word of encouragement.

Summary

The eating window is the period of time that you are allowed to indulge in foods and one that precedes a period of fasting. The eating window comes around on a cycle, and you should adhere to it by only eating when the window opens and abstaining from food the rest of the time. Intermittent fasting doesn't restrict the consumption of certain foods as is common for other weight loss methods such as fad diets. To boost the effectiveness of your fast, your diet should be balanced, which means it should include foods rich in minerals and vitamins. There also should be fruits and vegetables. Discipline is very important when it comes to fasting. It's what keeps you going when your body protests hunger. The most important step toward developing discipline is to first prepare mentally for the fast. Another way of developing discipline is by having a strong support system.

Part 3: Targeted Fasting for Your Body Type

Chapter 10: Fasting For Weight Loss

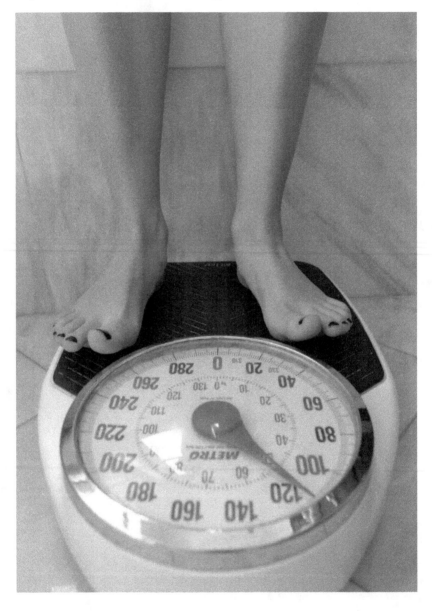

Why You'll Lose Weight through Fasting

Some of the methods of losing weight include fad diets, exercising, and supplements. However, these methods are not very effective, and in most cases, they cannot solve obesity on their own.

Fasting is easily the best method of not only reducing weight but also eliminating the stubborn lower-stomach fat. But why is it so?

First off, fasting optimizes the biological functions of your body. Fasting allows you to ease the load on your digestive system. The spare energy goes toward optimizing your physiological functions. For instance, improved digestion streamlines your bowel movement too. This efficacy in the physiological functions creates a compounding effect that leads to the shedding of dead weight, thus reducing an individual's weight and actually stabilizing it.

Another way in which fasting promotes weight loss is through cell autophagy. A dry fast is particularly what triggers cell autophagy. When the body uses up all its water, it now starts digesting the weak and damaged cells to provide water for the body cells that are in a much better state. Autophagy helps in eliminating dead and weak cells thereby making a person lighter.

Fasting plays a critical role in improving the metabolic health of an individual. With improved metabolism, the body can crunch more calories, and thus the individual's weight goes down.

Fasting improves insulin sensitivity. This helps the body to convert more sugars into energy. The body uses more calories, and as a result, there's a loss of weight.

In most obese people, the communication between their brain and ghrelin cells is warped, which makes them experience hunger all the time, even when they are full. Fasting helps remedy this problem, and obese people start receiving accurate signals when they are hungry.

Step-By-Step Process of Losing Weight through Fasting

- **Checkup**

First off, make sure that your body is in a condition that allows you to fast. Some of the people who are discouraged from the practice include pregnant women, nursing women, infants, sufferers of late-stage terminal illnesses, and those who are recovering from surgery.

- **Water**

Your body will respond to food deprivation by secreting acids and enzymes, and for that reason, always start your fast with consuming water. Regular water consumption will flush out the toxins and will also ease you from stomach pain.

- **Eating window**

Desist from food for at least 16 hours and then take a meal of your choice. The ideal eating window should be around eight hours. During this eight hour break, you are free to indulge. However, you must take care not to consume unhealthy foods. They will just neutralize your fasting efforts. Also, mind the portions. Simply because you have eight hours to feed doesn't mean you should fill up that period with food only.

- **Exercise**

Taking aerobic exercises, in particular, will have a dramatic effect on your weight loss. Aerobic exercises act like a calorie furnace. Also, exercises will increase the toxins in your body, and for that reason, keep yourself hydrated.

- **Breaking the fast**

At the end of your fast, never go right back into "heavy eating," but rather ease your way back by first consuming lighter foods. It'd be prudent of you to make fasting a part of your lifestyle. The key thing is to go with works for you. Most people seem to prefer intermittent fasting because it can fit in most people's lives. Prolonged fasting should be done sparingly as it carries the risk of developing complications.

Summary

Fasting has a positive impact on the rate of metabolism. When the metabolism rate is high, the energy output of the body goes up, and thus more calories are used up. This creates a caloric deficit and subsequent weight loss. Fasting promotes cell autophagy. Autophagy is the process where weak and damaged body cells are digested by the body. The elimination of weak body cells helps in weight reduction. High insulin resistance makes it hard for the body cells to absorb the sugars in the blood. But fasting reduces insulin resistance so that the body will use less insulin to convert sugars into energy. Before you go on a fast, you should get medical clearance. Some of the people who shouldn't get into a fast include the terminally ill, pregnant women, nursing women, and people who are recovering from surgery. It is important to take water throughout the fast to flush out toxins and mitigate the effect of stomach acids.

Chapter 11: Fasting for Type 2 Diabetes

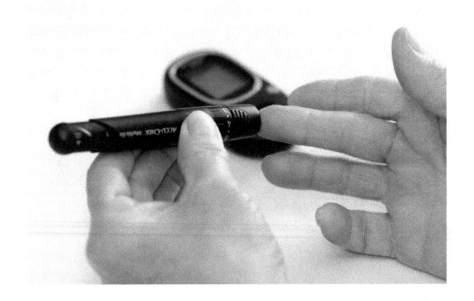

What is Type 2 Diabetes?

Type 2 diabetes is a disease that damages the ability of the pancreas to produce sufficient insulin. Insulin is the hormone produced by the pancreas, and its main function is to regulate the conversion of glucose into energy. The body cells of people who have type 2 diabetes are insensitive to insulin, and as such, they experience difficulty in converting sugars into energy. This condition is known as insulin resistance. It is characterized by the production of higher amounts of insulin, but the body cannot absorb it.

As to the origin of type 2 diabetes, scientists have established that it is genetic. The disease is handed down to progeny. Another leading cause of type 2 diabetes is obesity. Overweight people are much more likely to develop insulin resistance. There's a link between childhood obesity and development of type 2 diabetes in adulthood.

Another contributing factor is a metabolic syndrome. High insulin resistance is a result of increased blood pressure and cholesterol. Excessive sugars produced by the liver may also be a trigger.

The symptoms of type 2 diabetes cover a wide range. They include thirst, frequent peeing, hazy vision, irritability, tiredness, and yeast infections.

The risk of developing type 2 diabetes can be greatly minimized by taking the following actions:

Losing weight. Weight loss improves insulin sensitivity, and thus the buildup of insulin in the blood is eliminated. Also, there's more conversion of sugars into energy.

Balanced diet. You should consume foods that are sources of minerals and vitamins. Increase your intake of fruits and vegetables. Minimize your consumption of sugars and red meat.

The Role of Insulin in the Body

The insulin hormone is produced by the pancreas. Its key role is to regulate blood sugar. Increased insulin resistance might lead to type 2 diabetes. Insulin plays the critical role of facilitating absorption of sugars into body cells. In this way, insulin helps to reduce the blood sugar level. Another important role of insulin is to modify the activity of enzymes. The enzymes are secreted by the body when there's food in the stomach. Insulin regulates the activity of enzymes.

Insulin helps the body recover quickly. When your body is recovering from an injury or illness, insulin plays a critical role in speeding up the healing process by transporting amino acids to cells.

Insulin promotes gut flora and thus improves gut health. This improves bowel movement. Insulin also improves the excretion of harmful substances like sodium.

Insulin promotes brain health. It improves brain clarity by providing the essential nutrients to the brain.

Insulin plays a key role in determining the metabolism rate of the body. In instances of high insulin sensitivity, the blood glucose is easily absorbed into the cells, making for a high metabolic rate. But in instances of low insulin sensitivity, the process of converting sugars into energy becomes hard, and, consequently, there is a low metabolic rate.

Insulin is very important in the optimal functioning of your body. Some of the factors that improve the production of the insulin hormone are having a balanced diet, improving your brain health, having quality sleep, exercising, and staying in a pollution-free environment.

How Diabetes Affects both Production and Usage of Insulin

Diabetes is a major lifestyle disease all over the world. A person who has diabetes either cannot produce sufficient insulin, or their body cells are insensitive to insulin. Diabetes is broadly classified into two types: type 1 and type 2.

People who suffer from type 1 diabetes produce little to no insulin. This slows down the rate of conversion of sugars into energy. A low level of insulin is mainly a result of the immune system attacking the pancreas and curtailing its ability to produce sufficient insulin. Also, low insulin levels might be a result of weakened and damaged body cells. Type 1 diabetes commonly affects young people. One of the corrective measures is to administer insulin through injections.

Symptoms of type 1 diabetes include dehydration, constant urge to urinate, hunger (even after eating), unexplained weight loss, blurry vision, exhaustion, and bad moods.

Type 2 diabetes is the most common form of diabetes. People who suffer from type 2 diabetes have a high insulin resistance. Their body cells are averse to insulin. Types 2 diabetes is treated by increasing insulin sensitivity.

Symptoms of type 2 diabetes include tiredness, never-ending thirst, constant urge to pee, irritability, weak immune, and shivering.

The pancreas is the organ that produces insulin. When we consume food, blood sugar rises. The pancreas releases insulin to facilitate the conversion of sugars into energy. But someone who suffers from diabetes either lacks sufficient insulin or their body cannot use the released insulin. This results in increased blood sugar levels. This scenario presents risks such as the development of heart disease and stroke.

How Blood Sugar Responds To Fasting

A carbohydrate metabolism test is crucial in determining how blood sugar responds to fasting. The test is conducted on diabetics. During a fast, the levels of plasma glucose go up. People with diabetes either cannot produce sufficient insulin, or their bodies are resistant to insulin. Non-diabetics, though, produce insulin that brings down the levels of glucose through absorption.

Diet greatly affects the blood sugar rate-of-increase. For instance, a big serving of food will trigger a high level of blood sugar, and sugar-laden foods like cake, bread, and fries will also increase the blood sugar level.

People with type 1 diabetes lack sufficient insulin because their immune system attacks the pancreas, while people with type 2 diabetes are insensitive to insulin. So in both cases, there is a high level of blood sugar.

The levels of blood glucose during fasting give us insight into how the cells respond to blood sugar. A high level of blood glucose is indicative of the body's ability to lower blood glucose, and the conclusion might be either high insulin resistance or insufficient insulin production. Prolonged fasting has the effect of minimizing blood glucose levels. The sugars in the blood get used up, albeit slowly.

There are two methods of testing the level of blood sugar: the traditional blood sugar test, and the glycosylated hemoglobin (HbAlc). The glycosylated hemoglobin test is for checking how blood glucose has been changing. The traditional method of checking blood sugar involves daily tests which may be conducted by the affected person.

Developing Your Fasting Regimen

There are some fasting regimens. All of them have their pros and cons. They are only as good as the person trying to follow them. During fasts, it is recommended to take water to flush out toxins and also to mitigate hunger. However, if you want to improve the success rate of your fast, you might consider dry fasts, where you don't consume any fluid.

You may perform a fast for as short a time as a couple of hours or as long as a full week (and maybe even more, depending on your stamina). However, if your goal is to lose weight, then shorter fasts are more effective. For instance, intermittent fasting is many times more fruitful than prolonged fasting, but ultimately, you get to choose what you feel will work for you.

Short fasts allow you to go through a cycle of fasting and eating windows. You start by creating a plan in which you detail your period of fasting and when your eating window opens. During the eating window, it is advisable to consume unprocessed foods and avoid sugar-laden foods. This will boost your insulin sensitivity.

Long fasts have their benefits too, but on the whole, they are much less rewarding than short fasts. The strain associated with long fasts make you susceptible to infections and might, in the worst case scenario, rewire your physiological functions.

Things to Incorporate to Make Fasting Safe for Diabetics

When a diabetic goes on a fast, their body secretes the glucagon hormone, which leads to a spike in the blood sugar level. Thus, a diabetic should start by informing themselves properly before they deprive themselves of food.

The first thing is to determine whether they are fit to fast. A diabetic person should seek medical clearance before they attempt fasting. A person with advanced diabetes will have a low blood sugar level. If they go on a fast, they risk falling into a coma. A medical professional offers the best counsel as to how to conduct the fast and for how long.

For type 1 diabetics, it is important to have a test kit to observe the fluctuation of blood sugar throughout the fast. This helps in tweaking the fast or deciding whether to call it off.

Another safety measure is to have a confidant know of their fasting. The psycho-social support offered by a confidant would keep them going. The confidant should be someone in their close proximity that can monitor their progress.

Diabetics should indulge in a balanced diet during their eating window. A balanced diet comprises of foods rich in minerals and vitamins. One common thing that fasting induces is cravings. Fast foods, for instance, are sugar-laden and they have no real nutritional value. Indulging in fast foods during eating windows only negates the effectiveness of the fast.

A diabetic should know when to quit and how to quit. If there is a massive fluctuation of blood glucose, or if a complication develops, then that's a hint to quit. Towards the end of the fast, a diabetic should consume light meals first, and then transition back to their normal eating patterns.

Role of Supplements

A supplement is a substance that enhances the food that a person eats. The common types of ingredients in supplements include vitamins, minerals, botanicals, amino acids, enzymes, organ tissues, and glandulars. The supplements are critical in optimizing nutritional value of food. The water-soluble ingredients of supplements are metabolized and eliminated from the body same day, while fat-soluble elements may be stored in the body for several days or even weeks. Supplements may be taken on either a daily basis or alternately—depending on the elements they provide to the body. One should always seek the guidance of a medical professional about the number of supplements to consume.

Supplements are not as critical during short fasts as they are in prolonged fasts. The body is a store of many nutritional elements, and fasting induces the body to tap into its reservoirs, but it is still important to take supplements to discourage nutrition deficiency. Fat-soluble vitamins need to be taken alongside fats to make for easy absorption. They include vitamin A, vitamin D, vitamin E, and vitamin K. They are kept in body cells too. Water-soluble vitamins are eliminated on the same day, especially if your body is well hydrated. Water-soluble vitamins include B3, B2, B1, and acids. If you have a poor diet, water-soluble vitamins are stable sources of nutrition.

The primary function of supplements is to improve the nutritional value of a person's diet by supplying vital elements that are not easily accessible. Taking supplements while on a fast helps mitigate the side effects of fasting such as headaches and cramps.

Types of Supplements that Stabilize Electrolytes

Sodium. The intake of Sodium is dependent upon your level of physical activity. Generally, if you engage in tougher physical exercises, you should take a high dose. Sodium is vital in eliminating cramps and various pains in the body.

Potassium. This supplement is vital for the optimal functioning of the heart. Potassium deficiency is normally accompanied by problems such as increased heartbeat and blood pressure. Potassium also helps in the flow of blood. A person with potassium deficiency is bound to experience exhaustion and constant lethargic feeling.

Magnesium. People who are lacking in this vital nutrient experience a range of problems like low energy, anxiety, insomnia, indigestion, muscle aches, poor heart health, and migraines. Magnesium supplements help your body absorb magnesium at a higher rate. Magnesium should be taken alongside food as opposed to plainly for maximum health benefit.

Zinc. This supplement is very crucial in improving the health of an individual. It regulates appetite, improves taste, promotes weight loss, minimizes hair loss, mitigates digestive problems, and cures chronic fatigue. Additionally, zinc improves nerve health and boosts testosterone. Zinc, too, should be consumed alongside other meals for maximum health benefits.

Calcium. This supplement helps in strengthening the musculoskeletal frame of an individual, heart health, and reduces the risk of developing ailments like cancer and diabetes. Calcium and magnesium should be taken at separate times to avoid stunted absorption rates.

Iodine. Iodine is crucial in improving thyroid health. The thyroid gland secretes hormones that play a vital role in the basal metabolic rate.

How to Keep Insulin Levels Low

This hormone produced by the pancreas facilitates the absorption of sugars into body cells. The insulin levels should be stable for optimum metabolism to take place. High levels of insulin might lead to serious complications like high blood pressure. Someone with a high blood glucose level needs to lower their blood sugar level, else they may suffer serious health complications. Here are some of the ways to keep insulin levels low.

Diet. Your diet will have a direct impact on your blood sugar levels. Sugary, fat-laden foods will raise your blood glucose through the roof. On the other hand, a low-carb diet will help keep your blood glucose levels down.

Portion. There is a direct correlation between the portion of your food and your blood sugar levels. A giant portion of your favorite dish will lead to a surge in blood glucose. On the other hand, a small portion will keep your blood sugar stable. Bearing this in mind, you should aim to take small portions of food, as they minimize the fluctuation of blood glucose levels.

Exercise regularly. You can bring the high blood sugar levels down through exercise. When you exercise, your body powers your activities with the glucose in your blood. So exercises—and in particular, aerobics—can lead to low blood glucose levels.

Drink water constantly. Staying hydrated is also important in keeping the blood sugar level down. Water will flush out toxins and help streamline your metabolism.

Avoid alcohol. Alcohol not only lowers your inhibitions and makes you indulge in unhealthy foods like fries and roast meat, but it is also calorie-packed. If you aim to minimize your blood sugar, restrict your alcohol intake or drop it altogether.

What Causes Insulin Resistance?

Insulin is produced by the pancreas, and its work is to facilitate absorption of glucose into body cells. Insulin resistance is a condition where body cells are insensitive to insulin. For that reason, the rate of conversion of sugars into energy is affected. What are some of the causes of this condition?

Obesity. Most obese people have a ton of toxic elements stashed in their body. The combination of high blood sugar levels and toxic elements promote cellular inflammation. These cells naturally become insulin resistant.

Inactivity. Insulin resistance is common in people who hardly ever move their limbs. They don't perform any physical activity, so their energy requirement (output) is minimal. This creates some sort of "cell apathy" and promotes insulin resistance.

Sleep apnea. This is a sleep disorder characterized by faulty breathing. People who suffer from sleep apnea snore loudly and also feel tired after a night's sleep. Studies have shown a link between sleep apnea and development of insulin resistance in body cells.

High blood pressure. High blood pressure or hypertension is a degenerative medical issue where the blood pressure in blood vessels is more than 140/90 mmHg. Hypertension makes the heart's task of pumping out blood more difficult and may contribute to complications such as atherosclerosis, stroke, and kidney disease. Studies have shown a correlation between people with high blood pressure and the development of insulin resistance.

Smoking. The habit of smoking can give you many health complications. One of them is the risk of cancer development. Additionally, smoking seems to promote insulin resistance.

How Insulin Resistance Affects the Body

Insulin resistance makes it hard for the body cells to absorb sugars, which leads to high blood glucose levels. Some of the causes of insulin resistance include obesity, poor diet, sleep disorders, and sedentary lifestyle.

The American Diabetes Association (ADA) has stated that there is a 70% chance for people with insulin resistance to develop type 2 diabetes if they don't change their habits.

Insulin resistance may trigger the development of acanthosis nigricans, a skin condition in which dark spots cover parts of the body, especially the neck region.

Insulin resistance enhances weight gain, because it slows down base metabolism, causing a surge of blood sugar levels. Insulin carries off the excess blood sugar into fat stores, and thus, the person gains weight.

Insulin resistance promotes high blood pressure. The elevated blood glucose levels cause the heart to have to struggle with pumping more blood, causing high blood pressure.

Insulin resistance causes constant thirst and hunger pangs. Insulin resistance promotes the miscommunication between brain receptors and body cells. Thus, the brain activates the hunger hormone and makes the person eternally hungry. If not corrected, this leads to overeating and eventually chronic obesity.

Insulin resistance weakens the body. Insulin resistance leads to low energy output. And for that reason, the body doesn't have a lot of energy to use up, which makes the person feel (and look) weak.

Insulin resistance makes you urinate frequently; the condition affects the efficiency of physiological functions, and one of the results is a constant need to urinate.

Insulin resistance makes the body more susceptible to attack by diseases.

The Role of Amylin

Amylin is a protein hormone. It is produced by the pancreas alongside insulin. Amylin helps in glycemic control by promoting the slow emptying of the gastric and giving feelings of satisfaction. Amylin discourages the upsurge of blood glucose levels.

Amylin is part of the endocrine system, and it plays a critical role in glycemic control. The hormone is secreted by the pancreas, and its main function is to slow down the rate of appearance of nutritional elements in the plasma. It complements insulin.

Amylin and Insulin are secreted in a ratio of 1:100. Amylin delays gastric emptying and decreases the concentration of glucose in the plasma, whereas insulin facilitates absorption of sugars into cells. Diabetic people lack this hormone.

The amylin hormone can coalesce and create amyloid fibers, which may help in destroying diabetes. Amylin is secreted when there is the stimulus of nutrition in the blood. Unlike insulin, it is not purged in the liver but by renal metabolism.

Recent studies have shown the effect of amylin on the metabolism of glucose. In rats, amylin promoted insulin resistance.

Amylin slows down the food movement through the gut. As the food stays longer in the stomach, the rate of conversion of these foods to sugars will be slower.

Amylin also prevents the secretion of glucagon. Glucagon causes a surge in blood sugar level. Amylin prevents the inappropriate secretion of glucagon, which might cause a post-meal spike in blood sugar.

Amylin enhances the feeling of satiety. By reducing appetite, amylin ensures low blood glucose levels.

How Amylin Deficiency Affects Your Body

Amylin regulates the concentration of glucose in the blood by preventing the secretion of glucagon and slowing down the movement of food along the gut. People who suffer from diabetes have an amylin deficiency that causes excessive amounts of glucose to flow into the blood.

Increased insulin. A deficiency in amylin causes an extreme surge in blood glucose levels. To mitigate this spike, the pancreas secretes more insulin to help in the absorption of sugars into body cells. Increased levels of insulin in the blood might lead to complications.

Insulin resistance. Amylin deficiency eventually leads to high blood glucose levels. This might cause insulin resistance in body cells and, in worst case scenarios, it might trigger the immune system to attack the pancreas. High insulin levels in the blood might trigger memory loss and might even induce a coma.

Diabetes. Amylin deficiency leads to the overproduction of insulin, which, in the long run, impairs the pancreas. When the normal working of the pancreas is damaged, diabetes may develop.

Weight gain. Amylin deficiency promotes insulin resistance. When body cells become insensitive to insulin, there is less sugar converted into energy. So, the blood glucose level remains high. Insulin is responsible for carrying off these sugars to be stored as fats. Instead of these sugars being used as energy, they end up being stored as fat in the cells, which is the start of weight gain.

Headache. Thanks to insulin resistance, the body cells lack a reliable source of energy, which causes the body to switch to burning fats as an alternative energy source. One of the side effects of this process is normally headache and nausea.

The Insulin Resistance Diet

Insulin resistance causes slower absorption of sugars into body cells. This condition is rampant in obese people and diabetics. It is projected that the number of diabetics in the next 20 years will be over 320 million. This indicates a very worrying trend of diabetes. One of the things we can do to fight against diabetes is to improve our diet. Studies have shown that weight loss is a very effective means of minimizing insulin resistance. Here are the components of an insulin resistant diet:

Low carbs. Food high in carbs are responsible for blood sugar spikes. High levels of blood glucose promote insulin resistance. To ensure a stable blood glucose level, you should stick to low-carb foods.

Avoid sugary drinks. The American Diabetes Association advises against consumption of sugary drinks. These drinks with high sugar content include fruit juice, corn syrup, and other concentrates. Sugary drinks have a high sugar content, and they spike blood sugar levels. So, it'd be prudent to stay away from sugary drinks.

More fiber. Fiber is important in reducing the blood glucose levels. It improves the digestive health and improves blood circulation.

Healthy fats. Monounsaturated fats are very critical in improving heart health and regulating insulin levels.

Protein. Studies show that dietary protein is beneficial for people who suffer from diabetes. Regular consumption of protein is important for muscle growth and bone mass.

Size. Instead of taking large servings of a meal, opt for smaller portions of food, so that your post-meal blood glucose levels may be stable.

The Best Food for Diabetics

Diabetics don't have the luxury of eating any food they might want. For instance, sugar-laden foods and high-fat foods would spike their blood sugar levels and worsen the condition. They should instead stick to foods that are sources of minerals and vitamins. Foods like:

Fish. Fish is an important source of omega-3 fatty acids. These fatty acids are especially great for people with heart health complications and those who are at risk of stroke. Omega three fatty acids also protect your blood vessels, as well as reduce inflammation. Studies show that people who consume fish on the regular have better heart health than those who don't.

Greens. They are very nutritious and have low calories. Leafy greens like kale and spinach are excellent sources of minerals and vitamins. Leafy greens reduce inflammation markers, as well improve blood pressure. They are also high in antioxidants.

Eggs. The good old egg has been abused at the hands of intellectual conmen who have long said, albeit incorrectly, that eggs are bad. Eggs are excellent for reducing heart disease complications and also decreasing inflammation markers. Regular consumption of eggs improves cholesterol and blood glucose levels.

Chia seeds. They are high in fiber, and this fiber is critical in lowering blood glucose levels as well as in slowing down the rate of movement of food along the gut.

Nuts. Nuts are both tasty and healthy. They are great sources of fiber and are low in carbs. Regular consumption improves heart health and reduces inflammation and improves blood circulation.

Summary

Type 2 diabetes is a degenerative disease that impairs the ability of the pancreas to produce insulin. The hormone insulin is produced by the pancreas, and its main function is to regulate the conversion of glucose to energy. The risk of developing diabetes can be greatly minimized by taking the two steps: losing weight and having a balanced diet. The number of people with diabetes is at an all-time high, and people in both developed and poor countries are battling the disease. Symptoms of type 2 diabetes include tiredness, never-ending thirst, the constant urge to pee, irritability, weak immune system, and shivering. A carbohydrate metabolism test determines how blood sugar reacts to fasting. During a fast, blood sugar levels go up. Supplements are necessary for supplying important nutrients that may not be in the diet. The intake of supplements should be daily for optimum results. The important supplements include sodium, potassium, magnesium, zinc, calcium, and iodine. These are some of the measures to take to keep insulin levels low: have a strict diet, consume small portions, exercise regularly, and drink water constantly.

Chapter 12: Fasting For Heart Health

How Fasting Improves Your Heart's Health

Numerous studies have shown that fasting has a positive impact on heart health. Many people who have gone on a fast have reported feeling energetic and livelier afterward, which could be attributed to improved blood flow and general heart health. However, you need to fast consistently to achieve results.

Improves your heartbeat. When you go on a fast, your body is free from the digestion load, and so it channels that energy into optimizing your physiological functions. Your heart stands to gain from the optimized body functions, especially improving your heartbeat.

Improves blood pressure. Studies show that fasting has a positive impact on blood pressure. The rate of blood pressure is affected by factors like weight gain and obesity. But since fasting helps in weight loss, it has the extended advantage of lowering blood pressure, which improves the overall heart health.

Reduces cholesterol. Regularly fasting helps in lowering bad cholesterol. Also, controlled fasting increases the base metabolic rate.

Improved blood vessel health. Fasting is critical in improving the health of blood vessels. When blood vessels are subjected to high blood pressure, they slowly start to wear out, and might eventually burst up—which could be fatal, especially in the case of arteries. But fasting helps reduce blood pressure and bad cholesterol. The result is improved blood flow and overall heart health.

Autophagy. Regular dry fasts trigger the body to digest its weak and damaged cells in a process known as autophagy. Cell autophagy is very crucial because it helps eliminate old and damaged cells and creates room for new cells. With a new batch of cells to work with, the heart health is given a tremendous boost.

Summary

Fasting has been shown to improve the health of the heart. When you are fasting, your body reserves energy that would have gone into digestion for purposes of improving the heart health. It can execute its physiological functions much better. Fasting has also been shown to improve blood pressure. Fasting helps reduce obesity and reduces weight gain. This causes massive improvement in blood pressure. Fasting also plays a critical role in reducing cholesterol. Bad cholesterol increases the rate of developing heart disease. Also, controlled fasting increases the base metabolic rate. Fasting also improves the health of blood vessels. High blood pressure might cause blood vessels to wear out slowly, but fasting has a restorative effect on the blood vessels. Fasting also allows the body to digest its weak cells and make room for new and powerful body cells.

Chapter 13: The General Results of Fasting

Positive Effects of Fasting

You will get varied results depending on your preferred method of fasting, whether it's intermittent fasting, alternate-day, or prolonged fasting. These are some of the positive effects of fasting:

Weight loss. Fasting is an efficient way of losing weight. A study in 2015 showed that alternate fasting for a week resulted in weight loss of up to seven percent. When your body uses up the glucose in your blood, it now turns to the fat reserves to power its bodily functions. This helps in achieving weight loss.

Release of the human growth hormone. The human growth hormone promotes the growth of muscles and reduces obesity. Fasting triggers the secretion of the human growth hormone. This hormone is very crucial in building your body cells.

Improves insulin sensitivity. Low insulin sensitivity restricts the absorption of sugars into body cells. This might lead to complications such as chronic weight gain. Fasting leads to high insulin sensitivity that helps in absorption of sugars into body cells.

Normalizes ghrelin levels. Ghrelin is the hunger hormone which sends out hunger signals. Most obese people have abnormal ghrelin hormone levels that keep them in a perpetual state of hunger. Fasting, however, remedies this situation by normalizing ghrelin hormone levels, and thus you can receive accurate signals about hunger.

Lowers triglyceride levels. Depriving yourself of food for a set period of time has the effect of lowering bad cholesterol, and in the process, triglycerides are reduced.

Slows down aging. Many studies have shown the link between fasting and increased longevity in animals. Fasting allows the body to cleanse itself, promotes cell autophagy, and in the long run, lengthens lifespan.

Negative Effects of Fasting

As much as fasting is a practice with many benefits, admittedly there is a dark side too. These are some of the negative effects of fasting:

Strained body. A prolonged fast might put a big deal of a strain on your body. This may alter—albeit slightly—the normal processes of your body. A prolonged fast might slow down the effectiveness of your body as the body adapts to survive on too little energy.

Headaches. Headaches are common during fasts, especially at the start. The headache is normally a response of the brain to diminished blood glucose levels that force the body to switch to burning fats as a source of energy.

Low blood pressure. Fasting is a major cause of low blood pressure. Low blood pressure slows down the conversion of sugars into energy. This may lead to complications such as temporary blindness and, in extreme cases, can induce a coma.

Eating disorders. For someone who's too eager, it is easy to abuse fasting and turn it into an eating disorder. The main aim of fasting is to improve health, but starving yourself and having an eating disorder is anything but healthy. Some of the eating disorders that people who fast are at risk of developing include anorexia and bulimia.

Cravings. The hunger triggered by fasting might cause us to overcompensate. We may develop cravings for fast foods and other unhealthy foods. During our eating window, we may find ourselves consuming a lot of unhealthy foods, under the delusion that the fast will override that.

Summary

Weight loss is one of the main benefits of fasting. When you fast, your blood glucose is diminished, and this forces your body to turn to fats as an alternative source of energy. Fasting also promotes the production of the human growth hormone. This is the hormone responsible for muscle growth. Fasting also improves insulin sensitivity. Low insulin sensitivity impairs the body's ability to convert sugars into energy. Fasting also leads to high insulin sensitivity that helps in the absorption of sugars into body cells. Fasting also helps normalize ghrelin levels. The ghrelin hormone is known as the hunger hormone. Most obese people have abnormally high ghrelin levels that give incorrect hunger signals and make the obese person perpetually hungry. Fasting helps in correcting this problem, and the obese person starts to receive accurate signals. The negative effects of fasting include straining the body, headaches, low blood pressure, and eating disorders.

Part 4: Important Factors that Improve the Quality of Fasting

Chapter 14: Nutrition

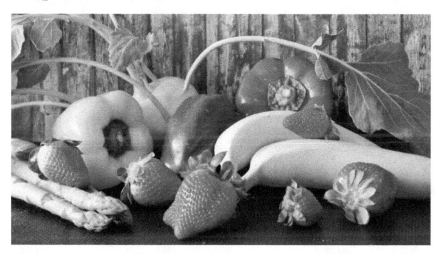

What Constitutes Good Nutrition?

Good nutrition implies a diet that contains all the required and important nutrients in appropriate proportions. When you fail to observe good nutrition, you risk developing complications from certain nutrient deficiencies. A good nutrition shouldn't be a one-off thing, but it should be a part of your lifestyle.

A great nutrition minimizes the risk of developing health complications such as diabetes, heart disease, and chronic weight gain. Here are the most important constituents of great nutrition:

- **Protein**

This nutrient is very important for muscle health, skin health, and hair. Also, it assists in the bodily reactions. Amino acids are essential for human growth and protein is stacked with amino acids. The best sources of protein include fish, eggs, and lentils.

- **Carbohydrates**

Carbohydrates are the main sources of energy for the body. They provide sugars that are converted into energy. There are two classes of carbohydrates: simple and complex. Simple carbohydrates are digested easily, and complex carbohydrates take time. Fruits and grains are some of the main sources of simple carbohydrates whereas beans and vegetables are sources of complex carbohydrates. For proper digestion, dietary fiber (carbohydrate) is needed. Men need a daily intake of 30 grams of fiber and women need 24 grams. Important sources of dietary fiber include legumes and whole grains.

- **Fats**

Fats play an essential role in health improvement. Both monounsaturated and polyunsaturated fats are healthy. Sources of monounsaturated fats include avocados and nuts. As for polyunsaturated fats, seafood is a major source. Unhealthy fats include trans fats and saturated fats, mostly found in junk food.

- **Vitamins**

Vitamins A, B, C, D, E, and K are necessary for the body's optimal functioning. A deficiency in the important vitamins can lead to serious health complications and weakened immune system.

- **Minerals**

Calcium, iron, zinc, and iodine are some of the essential minerals. They are found in a variety of foods including vegetables, grains, and meats.

- **Water**

Most of the human body is composed of water. It is a very essential nutrient for the proper functioning of the body.

Why Good Nutrition Is Important
The main reason why people ensure that they have a good nutrition is to improve their health. A good nutrition is essentially about consuming foods that are rich in vitamins, minerals, and fats. So, here

are some of the reasons why good nutrition is vital.

Reduces risk of cancer. Good nutrition plays a vital role in optimizing your health. If you consume healthy food, you drastically reduce your chances of getting cancer, as many cancers are a result of bad lifestyle choices.

Reduces risk of developing high blood pressure. High blood pressure causes a strain on the heart. It also leads to the wearing and tearing of the blood vessels. Having good nutrition normalizes your blood pressure and thus improves your heart health.

Lowers cholesterol. Bad cholesterol leads to serious complications like heart disease. When you observe good nutrition that involves fruits and essential vitamins, the bad cholesterol is eliminated, thus improving the functioning of your body.

Increased energy. Bad food choices have a draining effect. However, nutritious foods replenish the body cells with vital nutrients, and thus the body is active. A nutritious diet is a key to improving productivity.

Improved immunity. Diseases are always looking for new victims. People who have a poor diet are bound to have a weak immune system. The weak immune system won't sufficiently protect them against attacks. On the other hand, people who consume a nutritious diet tend to have a strong immune system. This improved immunity keeps diseases at bay.

The Advantages of a High-Fat Diet

Many studies have shown that a low-carb, high-fat diet has many health benefits, including weight management, and reduced risk of diabetes, cancer, and Alzheimer's. A high-fat diet is characterized by low carbohydrate intake and high intake of fat. The low carbohydrate intake puts the body into ketosis, a condition that optimizes burning of fat and helps convert fat into ketone bodies that act as an energy source of the brain. These are some of the advantages of a high-fat diet:

Stronger immune system. Saturated fats are an ally of the immune system. They help fight off microbes, viruses, and fungi. Fats help in the fight against diseases. A great source of saturated fats includes butter and coconut.

Improves skin health and eyesight. When someone is lacking in fatty acids, they are likely to develop dry skin and eyes. Fatty acids help in improving skin elasticity and strengthening eyesight.

Lowers risk of heart disease. Saturated fats trigger production of good cholesterol, which is key in reducing the risk of heart disease. Saturated fats also help fight inflammation. A good source of saturated fats includes eggs and coconut oil.

Strong bones. Healthy fats improve the density of bones and thus minimize the risk of bone diseases. Fats promote healthy calcium metabolism. Fatty acids, too, play a critical role in minimizing the risk of bone complications such as osteoporosis.

Improves reproductive health. Fats play a critical role in the production of hormones that improve fertility in both men and women. A high-fat diet improves reproductive health and, in particular, the production of testosterone and estrogen.

Weight loss. A high-fat diet promotes high metabolism and, as a result, the body can crunch more calories, leading to weight loss.

Improved muscle gain. A high-fat diet promotes muscle gain. This is achieved through hormone production and speeding up cell recovery after strenuous exercise.

Role of Ketone Bodies

The three ketone bodies produced by the liver include acetoacetate, beta-hydroxybutyrate, and acetone. Ketone bodies are water-soluble, and it takes a blood or urine test to determine their levels.

Ketone bodies are oxidized in the mitochondria to provide energy. The heart uses fatty acids as fuel in normal circumstances, but during ketogenesis, it switches to ketone bodies. When the blood glucose levels are high, the body stores the excesses as fat. When you go for an extended period of time without eating, the blood glucose levels diminish. This triggers the body to convert fat into usable energy. Most body cells can utilize fatty acids, except the brain. The liver thus converts fats into ketone bodies and releases them into the blood to supply energy to the brain. When ketone bodies start to build up in the blood, problems might arise. An increase in the levels of acetone can induce acidosis, a condition where blood pH is lowered. Acidosis has a negative impact on most of the body cells, and in worst cases, it leads to death. With that in mind, it is prudent to replenish your body with carbohydrates as soon as ketosis kicks off. A person with type 1 diabetes is more susceptible to high levels of ketone bodies. For instance, when they fail to take an insulin shot, they will experience hypoglycemia. The combination of low blood glucose level and high glucagon level will cause the liver to produce ketone bodies at an alarming rate which might cause complications.

Benefits of the Ketogenic Diet

Here are some of the benefits associated with ketone bodies:

Treating Alzheimer's. Alzheimer's behaves in a way similar to diabetes. Essentially, it is the brain resisting insulin. Due to insulin resistance, the brain only gets minimal energy, which might cause the death of brain cells. However, ketone bodies are an alternative source of energy that the brain can utilize. Ketone bodies have been shown to prevent a buildup of compounds that enhance the development of Alzheimer.

Normalizes insulin production. Ketone bodies are only produced when blood glucose is low. For this reason, the pancreas stops pumping more insulin to aid in the absorption of sugars because the body has already switched into ketogenesis.

Regulates metabolism. Ketone bodies regulate metabolism through their effects on mitochondria. The mitochondria are the cells' power plants, and they respond better to energy from fats rather than glucose. In this sense, ketone bodies improve the functioning of the mitochondria.

Lowers hunger. When the body is utilizing ketone bodies, it seems that there's less of an urge to consume food. Ketogenesis regulates the hunger hormone. When a person is consuming fast foods, there is no end to the urge to take another serving. Eventually, this leads to weight gain.

Increases good cholesterol. The good cholesterol improves blood flow and the condition of your heart. Ketogenesis helps in the production of the good cholesterol and thus helps in improving heart health.

Improves brain health. Ketone bodies are especially effective as a source of energy for the brain. Many people who have practiced the ketone diet say that it improves their mental clarity and focus.

The Importance of a Well-Balanced Diet

When we talk about a balanced diet, we refer to a variety of foods that supply us with important nutrients such as protein, carbohydrates, healthy fats, vitamins, and minerals. So, what is the importance of a well-balanced diet?

Strengthens immune system. When you consume a diet that's rich in nutrients, your immune system will become stronger. This places your body in a far better place to fight disease vectors that might have otherwise overwhelmed your body's defense system.

Weight loss. In the past, obesity was a problem in only developed nations. Not anymore. Nowadays even poor people are struggling with obesity. This is partially due to fast foods being cheaper and more convenient. As you can imagine, obesity has become a crisis the world over. The open secret is that obesity can be mitigated through a balanced diet. A diet rich in nutritious elements will nourish your body and also regulate your appetite so that you don't fall into the temptation of eating unhealthy foods.

Mental health. People who observe a balanced diet are less likely to fall into bad moods and depression. The nutritious elements stabilize their emotions and enable them to be more resistant to the autosuggestions of their mind.

Skin health. Dry skin is often the result of a bad diet. When you have a balanced diet, your skin and hair are nourished, and it gives you a glow. Foods rich in vitamins and collagen improve skin elasticity.

Promotes growth. A balanced diet helps kids have a well-formed body as they transition into adults and it helps adults maintain a well-figured body.

Summary

A good nutrition is a diet that contains all the important nutrients in appropriate portions. You risk developing complications if you fail to follow a good nutrition. The risk of developing health complications is greatly minimized by a great nutrition. Protein is one of the most important elements of a good nutrition. It is important for muscle health, skin health and development of hair. Protein also plays a role in bodily reactions. Carbohydrates are the major source of energy. They provide glucose that the body cells use to power activities of the body. Fats also play an important role in improving health. Monounsaturated fats and polyunsaturated fats are especially healthy. Vitamins are necessary for the body to function optimally. Minerals and water are important too. People ensure that they have good nutrition to improve their health. They achieve this by consuming foods that are rich in nutritious elements. A high-fat diet promotes strong immunity, better eyesight, a lower risk of heart disease, and stronger bones.

Chapter 15: Exercise

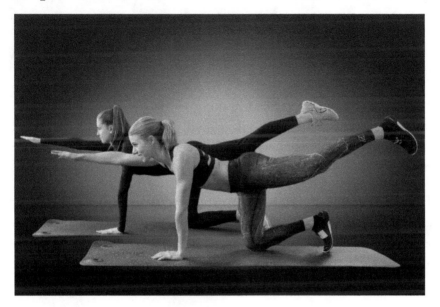

Pros of Exercising While Fasting

For the longest time, it was considered unhealthy to exercise while on a fast, but new evidence has shown that it is perfectly healthy to exercise even while you are fasting.

When you fast for health purposes, it shows that you are committed to improving your health and managing your weight. One of the ways you could get better results is by turning to physical exercise. A combination of intermittent fasting and physical exercise will burn up calories and help you reach your health goals in the shortest time possible.

The time of day that you exercise seems to affect the outcome. For instance, exercising in the morning right after you wake up promotes more weight loss than exercising at night. For intermittent fasting to be effective, you need to abstain from food for at least 16 hours.

When you exercise while on a fast, you speed up weight loss and optimize your health because of increased oxidation that promotes the growth of muscle cells.

It enriches your blood. Exercising has a positive effect on your breathing system and lung capacity. This helps in increasing the oxygen levels in your blood.

Exercising also improves heart health. Aerobic exercises, in particular, improve blood circulation and develop the stamina of the heart. Now, the blood pressure stabilizes and nutrients can spread to the whole body.

Exercising while on a fast improves your body's adaptability. It is never a good idea to idle around while on a fast, as it will trigger cravings. However, when you engage in physical activity, your body starts to adapt. It helps you create more stamina to endure your fast.

Best Exercises to Do

Exercising while fasting increases the rate of calorie burning. As a result, more weight is lost, and health is optimized in much less time. Here are the best exercises to perform while on a fast:

- **Aerobic exercise**

Aerobic exercise increases your heartbeat and breathing cycle. Aerobic exercise also improves lung capacity and heart health. Some of the benefits of aerobic exercise include improved mental health, minimized inflammation, lowered blood pressure, lowered blood sugar, and a minimized risk of heart disease, stroke, type 2 diabetes, and cancer. Aerobic exercises tend to be intense and easy to perform. Some examples of aerobic exercises include dancing, speed-walking, jogging, and cycling.

- **Strength training**

Strength training is important for muscle gain. People who perform strength training have more energy and keep their bodies at peak performance. Strength training improves your mental health, decreases blood sugar levels, enhances weight management, corrects posture, increases balance, and relieves pain in the back and joints. Strength training may be performed either in the gym or at home. Professional guidance depends on the exact exercise and equipment required. Strength training mostly takes the form of exercises such as pull-ups, push-ups, sit-ups, squats, and lunges. It is recommended to take breaks from strength training to allow muscle growth.

- **Stretching**

Stretching exercises are vital in improving the flexibility of a person. The exercises are designed to improve the strength and flexibility of tendons. Stretching exercises also improve the aesthetic quality of muscles. They also improve the circulation of blood and promote nourishment of all body cells.

- **Balance exercises**

Balance exercises promote agility. The exercises are designed to make your joints flexible. Balance exercises lead to improved focus and motor skills. The exercises include squats, sit-ups, and leg lifts.

Summary

Contrary to what people thought for the longest time, it is healthy to exercise while on a fast. A combination of exercise and fasting is a resource-intensive activity that makes your body burn more calories. Studies show that exercising in the morning has a far better outcome than exercising at night before bed. When you exercise while fasting, oxidation in cells promotes the growth of muscles. Exercising while on a fast also enriches your blood. The improved breathing cycle and lung capacity help in increasing the level of oxygen in the blood.

Exercising is vital in improving heart health and blood circulation. It is never a good idea to stay idle while you are on a fast. Your hunger will be magnified, and it might cause to break the fast. Some of the best exercises to do for maximum weight loss and health improvement include aerobic exercises, strength training, stretching and balance exercises.

Chapter 16: Having a Partner to Keep You in Check

Role of a Partner

Depriving yourself of food is by no means easy. If you have no experience, the temptation to slide back is real. In some instances, fasting might make you lapse into a worse state than before. This is especially after a small duration of fasting where the hunger is extreme, and then you are tempted into eating unhealthy foods, trapping you into eating them.

Having a partner to keep you in check is a good step, and if they are into fasting themselves, that's even better. Ideally, your partner should be someone that "understands" you. He or she will make fasting less taxing. They will be there to see your progress and offer constructive criticism when needed. As your fasting progresses, they will help you adjust accordingly or make tweaks, to go through the fast in the safest manner possible.

Your partner will hold you accountable for your fasting journey. Attaining health goals is no easy task. It takes dedication, discipline, and consistency. It's exactly why you need a partner to hold you accountable when you stray or when you fall back on your goals. A responsible partner will be interested in your gains (i.e., asking questions about your weight loss so far and wanting to know what your diet is like).

A partner is also important because you have someone to talk to about your journey. They can offer you psychosocial support in your moments of vulnerability. It makes a world of difference. And you will stick to your goals knowing that someone cares.

Traits to Look for in a Partner

Not everyone may qualify to be a partner to someone who's fasting.

The first thing to look out for is their opinion on the subject of fasting. Some people seem to think that fasting is a bad practice and a waste of time. Clearly, you wouldn't want such a person as your partner.

- **Patience**

Your partner should demonstrate patience. You cannot rush things while fasting. Sometimes, the results might take time, and in such situations, the last thing you want is someone on your neck, probably trashing your methods.

- **Observation skills**

A great partner must be a good observer. Their job is to spot loopholes that need to be closed, to assess situations, and to weigh overall progress. They need strong observation skills that will make them suitable for their positions. Also, remember that it is sometimes critical to call off a fast. Maybe you will be hard on yourself even when you are falling apart. An observant partner should notice the change and suggest that you stop.

- **Communication skills**

They should have good communication skills. What good is it to know something and not express it in a timely and appropriate fashion? A great partner should be very communicative and should express him/herself in an elaborate manner.

- **Knowledgeable**

A good partner should be knowledgeable. They should have a working knowledge of the whole subject of fasting. During every step of the fast, they should have a mental picture of what's coming. This will strengthen your bond and together you can meet any challenge.

- **Respect**

They should be able to respect you, your methods, and also have self-respect. This creates an enabling environment.

Should You Join A Support Group?

When your brain floods you with hunger hormones during a fast, the temptation to quit is real. One of the methods to minimize your chances of quitting is to join a support group. This is ideally a group of people who have similar fasting pursuits as you. Now you have a family to keep you in check and boost your confidence.

A support network will allow you to cope and express your feelings and get connected with like-minded people. In times of vulnerability, others will come to your help. As other members share their experiences, you learn that you are not alone, and you even broaden your perspective and wisdom.

Support networks include people who are at various stages toward the common goal you all have. In times of conflict, you have ready help, and if you are at an advanced stage yourself, then you should offer help to those in need of it too. Support networks have non-judgmental environments and therapeutic effects.

The best support groups are those that foster frequent get-togethers. Ideally, the members should come from the same society, but that doesn't mean other kinds of support groups are necessary. For instance, you could join an online support network and be free to commune with your family at your convenience. Online support groups seem to be a thing nowadays. People from around the world with common goals are coming together to form support networks.

The most important thing when you join a support group is to become a giver rather than a taker. Or both. When everyone is interested in giving, you have a resourceful group of like-minded people.

Summary

People who are overwhelmed by the idea of staying without food should consider getting a partner. Your partner should help you cultivate a strong sense of discipline and stick to your routine. Ideally, your partner should be someone who understands you. He or she will help you get through fasting. A supportive partner is there to check your progress and offer constructive criticism when the occasion calls for it. He or she should be someone that you can open up to and express your fears and concerns. With the right partner, your fasting journey will be smooth and enjoyable. Your partner should be patient, observant, communicative, respectful, and knowledgeable. Joining a support group will help you come together with other like-minded people for a common goal. You are guaranteed of ready help and psychosocial support. The best support group to join should comprise of people from your local area, but it doesn't rule out joining even online support groups and communing with people from different parts of the world.

Chapter 17: Motivation

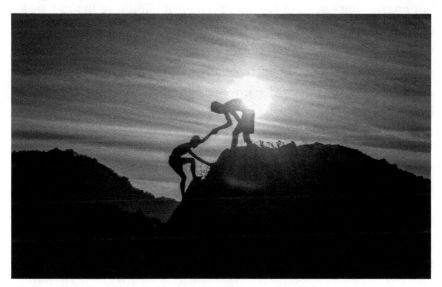

How to Stay Motivated Throughout Your Fast

Get a partner. If you go it alone, you are much more likely to forgive yourself and tweak the fast to suit you. For that reason, let there be a person to whom you are accountable. This person should put you in check and ensure that you follow the rules. Offer constructive criticism, and suggestions. A partner will help you stick to your routine. The ideal partner should be patient, empathetic, a good communicator, and knowledgeable about fasting. Let them share in your accomplishments as much as they have shared in your trials and struggle.

Seek knowledge. Being informed makes all the difference. You will know every possible outcome. You are aware of all the side effects of fasting and how to persist through the unpleasant experience instead of just quitting. Knowledge will help you optimize your fast and make you reap more benefits than anyone who had just deprived themselves of food. Being knowledgeable is important also in the sense that you are more aware of when to stop.

Set goals. Don't get into fasting with mental blindness. Instead, make an effort to set milestones. When you achieve a goal—for instance, when you hit your target weight—celebrate and then go back to reducing weight. Your brain responds to victory by making you feel confident. Now, you will have more confidence in your capacity to withstand hunger.

Develop positivity. A positive attitude makes all the difference. Keep reading about successful people who have achieved what you are looking for. Lockout all the negative energies that would derail you.

Record your progress. It is easy to underestimate yourself. As long as you keep going, the achievements will always be there. It's just a matter of recognizing them and celebrating.

How to Make Fasting Your Lifestyle

There are different approaches to fasting. You may fast every other day, once a week, or even a couple of times every month. In each instance, there are benefits.

But if you'd like to reap great benefits out of fasting, you should purposefully make it a daily ritual. Many people in the world today fast on a daily basis and have reported an increased quality of life.

The most common and most rewarding method is the 16:8 intermittent fasting. In this method, you fast for 16 hours in a day and then eat during the other 8 hours to complete the cycle.

Ideally, when you wake up, you should take a drink of water or black coffee and either exercise or just go on about your work. At around noon, your eating window opens, and you're free to have your meals up until 8 pm when the eating window closes.

During this eight-hour eating window, it is common to be tempted to overeat or indulge in unhealthy foods, thinking that the coming fast will "take care of that." Well, you must be careful not to fall into this temptation, or else your gains will be negated. Consume healthy and nutritious foods during the eating window and adhere to your 16-hour fast. The weight loss starts occurring in as short a span as a few days.

If you incorporate intermittent fasting into your lifestyle, the weight loss keeps going until you hit a stable weight where it plateaus. When fasting is your lifestyle, it makes your health improvement and weight loss permanent.

Summary

You need to take a few measures to stay motivated throughout the fast. One of the measures is to get a partner. A partner should hold you accountable and keep you in check so that you don't stray from the fasting routine. The ideal partner should be patient, empathetic, and a good communicator. Another way of motivating yourself is through seeking knowledge. As a knowledgeable person, you will be aware of all the responses that your body will give off. Knowledge will also help you optimize your fast and get the best possible results. Other ways to stay motivated throughout the fast include setting goals, developing positivity and recording your progress. If you make fasting part of your lifestyle, you stand to reap more benefits. The most common and most efficient fasting method is the 16:8, where you fast for 16 hours and then have an eating window of 8 hours.

Chapter 18: Foods for the Fast

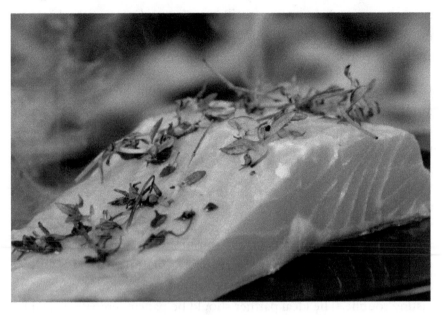

How Food Controls the Rate of the Success of Fasting

Depriving yourself of food is no easy task. Your body will tune up the hunger, and you will have to suppress the urge to feed. Not easy.

When you consume food, it is digested and released into the bloodstream as sugars. The pancreas secretes the hormone insulin to help in absorption of these sugars into body cells. When you stay for long without eating, there is no more food getting digested, and thus no more sugars getting released into the blood. The body soon runs out of the existing sugars and meets a crisis. The body is forced to switch to fats to provide energy for various physiological functions.

The foods that you eat have a massive impact on the efficacy of the fast. If you take light meals or small portions of food during the eating window, you will experience a higher degree of hunger during the fast.

On the other side, if you consume large amounts of food during your eating window, your hunger will not be as intense.

One of the tricks to reducing hunger during the fast is to consume foods that are high in dietary fiber. Such foods make you full for a long time and will thus minimize the unpleasant feeling triggered by hunger.

Consuming healthy foods during your eating window is important. Some people fall into the temptation of eating unhealthy foods or even eating too much, and the effect is negative.

Intermittent fasting is favored by many people because it doesn't restrict consumption of foods, unlike fad diets that insist on vegan meals or raw food.

The Worst Foods to Take During Fasting

If you want to speed up your weight loss and avoid lifestyle diseases, these are some of the foods to cut back on, or maybe stay away from:

Sugary drinks. The high dose of fructose in sugary drinks will cause an extreme surge of blood sugar levels. High amounts of this kind of sugar promote insulin resistance and liver disease. High levels of insulin resistance have a negative impact on the absorption of sugars into body cells. This creates the perfect recipe for the development of heart disease and diabetes.

Junk food. They might taste heavenly, but the ingredients of most junk foods come from hell. Junk foods have almost zero nutritional value. Fries are prepared using hydrogenated oil that contains trans fats. Studies have been made on trans fats, and the conclusion is that continued consumption of trans fats leads to heart complications and cancer.

Processed food. Most processed foods have a long shelf life thanks to a host of nasty chemicals poured into them. The processed foods are made durable to gain a commercial edge over organic products with a limited shelf life. Most processed foods are high in sugars, sodium, and have low fiber content and nutrients.

White bread and cakes. Baked goods tend to affect people with celiac disease, most especially. But more than that, most of these baked goods are stashed with processed ingredients—sugars and fats—and they are low on fiber. Most baked goods trigger abnormal surges in blood sugar levels and increase the risk of heart disease.

Alcohol. Studies show that alcohol induces inflammation on the liver. Excessive alcohol consumption will eliminate all the successes of your fast and promote weight gain and even development of diabetes.

Seed oils. Studies show that these oils are unnatural. They contain harmful fatty acids that increase the risk of developing heart complications.

The Best Foods to Take During Fasting
These are some of the best foods to indulge in while you fast to reach your important health goals:

Nuts. Nuts are rich in nutritional value. Almonds, Brazil nuts, lentils, oatmeal, etc. have properties that help in the production of good cholesterol. Good cholesterol promotes heart health. Nuts are excellent sources of vitamins and minerals. Oatmeal, in particular, is essential in normalizing blood glucose levels.

Fruits and greens. They are important sources of essential nutrients that improve both gut health and brain health. Broccoli is rich in phytonutrients that reduce the risk of heart complications and cancers. Apples contain antioxidants that eliminate harmful radicals. Kale contains the vital vitamin K. Blueberries are excellent sources of fiber and phytonutrients. Avocados are good sources of monounsaturated fats that lower bad cholesterol and improve heart health.

White meats. These are an excellent source of protein and fatty acids. Fish provide omega-3 fatty acids which improve heart health and stimulate muscle growth. Chicken is a great source of protein, and it promotes the growth of muscle cells.

Grains. They are excellent sources of protein and dietary fiber that will keep you full. Grains also help in improving heart health and normalizing blood pressure.

Eggs. Eggs are excellent sources of protein, and they tend to fill you up thus minimizing hunger levels.

Tubers. Foods such as potatoes and sweet potatoes are loaded with essential vitamins and carbohydrates.

Dairy. Dairy seems to reduce the risk of development of obesity and type 2 diabetes. Cheese and whole milk are excellent sources of protein and essential minerals that promote bone development.

Summary

When you go on a fast, your body increases the hunger levels in an attempt to pressure you to look for food. Staying without food for a long time causes the body to switch to fats as an alternative energy source. When the carbohydrates supplying energy to the brain are depleted, the liver produces ketone bodies to supply energy to the brain. The food you eat (and the portion) will impact your hunger levels during the fast. It is important to consume healthy foods during the eating window no matter how strong the temptation to stray is. Some of the worst foods that you can indulge in while fasting includes sugary drinks, junk foods, processed foods, white bread and cakes, alcohol, and seed oils. On the other hand, some of the best foods you can indulge in would be nuts, fruits and greens, white meat, grains, eggs, tubes, and dairy.

PART III

CHAPTER ONE

A WARNING

Everybody is different, making every habit different. That means that all these tips coming up are subjective. It's not something that will work for everybody. Another thing you need to be aware of is that your habit could be something more. I'm going to go over this possible problem quickly. Keep in mind this is not to cure or diagnose you with anything. If you think you may have a psychological disorder, as opposed to a bad habit, please seek medical attention.

For your information, a habit is defined as a settled or regular tendency or practice; especially one that is hard to give up.

OCD, obsessive compulsive disorder, can be confused as a habit. OCD can fall into four main categories;

- checking

- contamination/mental contamination

- hoarding

- ruminations/intrusive thoughts

OCD is diagnosed by when obsessions and compulsions:

- Consume excessive amounts of time

- Causes significant distress

- Interferes with daily functions

Your habit, itself, could be OCD, or your inability to break the habit, could be caused by OCD. An example of OCD being the habit would be hoarding. An example of OCD interfering your ability to break a habit would be intrusive thoughts. Now, when breaking a habit you will have intrusive thoughts, but they should just come and go. If your intrusive thoughts are constant and interfere with your life, then OCD could be a factor.

Other psychological disorders that could be confused with a habit are, eating disorders. Anorexia nervosa and bulimia nervosa are common eating disorders where people end up starving themselves or binging and purging. A lesser known eating disorder, which is the one most likely to be confused as a habit, is a binge-eating disorder.

With binge-eating disorder, people lose control of their eating habits. Unlike with bulimia nervosa, periods of binges are not followed by purging, which is why most people with binge-eating disorder are overweight. It is the top eating disorder in the US. Symptoms of binge-eating disorder are:

- Eating an unusually large amount of food in a specific amount of time

- Eating even when you're full or not hungry

- Eating fast during binge episodes

- Eating until you are uncomfortably full

- Eating alone or in secret to avoid embarrassment

- Feeling distressed, ashamed, or guilty when not eating

- Frequent dieting, possibly without weight loss

Chances are everybody can say that they have experienced one or more of these symptoms. For example, most holidays' people will over eat. That does not mean you have binge-eating disorder. Keep in mind disorders interrupt your everyday life, and happen constantly. If you just overeat when watching TV, or when you're bored, then you probably don't have a disorder. If you are concerned that you might, then please seek medical advice.

Make sure that if you think you have a disorder to see your doctor make sure. It's better to believe you have a disease than go around with an undiagnosed disorder. I want to make sure that you can live the life you deserve and making sure that your habit isn't something more serious is important.

CHAPTER TWO

A HISTORY OF HABITS

Imagine this; your alarm goes off. You slide out of bed and slump your way to the bathroom. You do your business and then hop in the shower. Once finished you brush your teeth before you get dressed. Once dressed you head to the kitchen to have your coffee and breakfast. Now, what just happened? You were on complete autopilot. You are so used to doing the same thing every morning you don't have to think about it. That is what a habit is.

Human beings are creatures of habit. We get into a routine, and we stick to it. Then it becomes a struggle to change.

Chances are your habits are caused by stress or boredom. You start doing things to distract your brain from the stress or boredom, giving you brain a brief moment of utopia.

Stress and boredom aren't just triggers for certain habits. They're triggers for most habits. Whether you have a problem with eating, smoking, biting your nails, or spending mindless hours on the computer, whatever it may be you're using the habit to suppress those emotions. There is a chance that a deeper issue causes the stress or boredom that is being felt.

Ask yourself, is there a belief or a reason you're holding onto this habit?

The key to overcoming a habit is to figure out what is causing it. Did something happen when you were younger? Do you believe something bad is going to happen if you stop?

That's why there is no one solution. Take the habit of smoking. According to the World Health Organization, more than one billion people smoke. Most of those people are smoking for different reasons. Some may smoke because they saw their parents smoke, or their friends. They may have started smoking as a way to cope with stress.

A Loop

Every habit begins with a psychological pattern. The habit loop is a three-part process. It begins with a trigger. The trigger tells you brain to go into automatic mode and let a behavior happen. The second part is the routine which is the actual habit itself. The last part is the reward. The reward is something your brain likes and helps it remember the loop in the future.

According to neuroscientists, habit-making behaviors are controlled in the basal ganglia. The basal ganglia are also the area of the brain that controls emotions, memories, and patterns. As stated above, a habit is a pattern.

Decisions are controlled in the prefrontal cortex. A habit starts as a behavior or decision, but the more you do it, the less the brain works. The decision-making part of your brain goes to sleep. That's what makes multitasking possible.

Good habits are programmed the same as bad habits are. A good habit, such as brushing your teeth, gets programmed by repetition just like smoking. Or learning to parallel park works the same as overeating.

The fact that they work the same is a good thing. That makes it easier for you to retrain your brain.

Problems

There are going to be problems when trying to break a habit, especially if your habit involves any stimulant. At that point, you're not just trying to stop the habit, but also working through the detox symptoms. For example, nicotine, via tobacco, is one of the most heavily consumed drugs in the world. In Australia, smoking is one of the biggest causes of, preventable, death, killing about 15,000 people per year. It's also one of the hardest to quit. Withdrawal from nicotine can cause insomnia, irritability, anxiety, and difficulty concentrating.

Slip-ups are inevitable, but if you're working to break a habit that involves any stimulating drug, it's going to be a lot harder. This could include smoking, drinking, even coffee. Keep this in the back of your mind so that you are prepared.

CHAPTER THREE

A HABITS HABITAT

Necessarily true. You can control your habits, but your environment plays a huge part of what you do on a daily basis. One of your brain's primary functions is to find and use patterns as shortcuts to process the information we're presented with on a daily basis.

In a study conducted on habits vs. intentions, researchers found that students that switched Universities were more likely to change their daily habits. Those habits were easier to change than they were for the control group because they weren't exposed to familiar daily cues. This can be seen in every bad habit that somebody has.

Eating Habits

Have you ever been driving home from work, not thinking about food, when you see your favorite fast food joint, and suddenly your start craving a cheeseburger? It's not your fault. Everybody experiences moments like that.

Our food environment is broken down into two categories; the atmosphere we encounter when eating, and how food is portioned. The cues vary from what's being eaten, its packaging or utensil size, and the amount of food. Think about when you eat out. You will undoubtedly receive a huge plate of food. You don't think you can eat it all, but then you end up cleaning your plate. Seeing an empty plate signals satiety in our brains.

Maybe eating at home will help you avoid these triggers. Not so fast.

Home plate sizes have increased 22% over the last century. Where you store your food also plays a large part in your eating habits, bringing new meaning to "Out of sight, out of mind."

Don't worry though. There are ways to overcome these triggers.

- First, choose smaller plates to use at home. It takes less food to fill up a small plate. You're eating less, but you're still cleaning your plate and making your brain happy.

- Another way is to pre-portion your food. Have everything portioned out into single servings.

- It also helps to focus on one thing at a time. When you're eating, only concentrate on eating. Try not to watch TV or the computer while you're eating.

- Most importantly learn the true signs of hunger and avoid mindless eating. This comes in handy when you're not in control of the food.

Smoking Habits

Environmental triggers for smokers can be harder to break than triggers for overeaters. According to the American Psychological Association is in an area associated with smoking can cause a smoker to have a craving. That means they could walk into a bar where there are no cigarettes, ashtrays, or other smokers, yet still, have a craving because they associate the setting with smoking.

Your regular daily routine could also cause triggers. Some people associate their morning cup of coffee with smoking. An easy fix for that is to keep yourself busy in the morning. Try to distract yourself from the craving. You can also trade your coffee out for tea or juice.

Most smokers smoke while driving making the car another common trigger. If you have cravings whenever you drive try singing along to the radio or a CD. You could also substitute smoking with chewing gum while driving.

Stress is another major trigger for smokers. Cigarettes have thousands of chemicals in them that trick your brain into thinking that they are helping relieve your stress. The key to overcoming the stress trigger is to find new ways to relieve your stress. Meditation and yoga are both good stress management techniques.

Drinking Habits

Stress and anxiety are big triggers for drinking. As I mentioned earlier, they are also the cause for most habits.

There are two main types of triggers; external and internal. External are people, places, or things that trigger you desire to drink. They are easier to avoid than internal triggers. Internal triggers are, as the name states, inner emotions that trigger your desire to drink.

A good way to figure out exactly what causes your triggers is to track them for a week. Keep a journal with you and every time you have the urge to drink, write down what happened or where you were that caused the urge.

Some simple ways to avoid external triggers are to keep little, to no alcohol, at home. Socially, try avoiding situations that involve drinking. You may feel guilty turning down invitations to go out with your friends, but just remember it's not forever. You only have to turn them down until your urges become more manageable.

It won't be possible to stay away from all triggers. Always remind yourself why you are making this change. Keep a list somewhere on your person that you can read when you have the urge to drink. Talk to an accountability partner. That's what they're there for. Distract yourself. Find something to do to keep your mind off your urge. Lastly, you could also ride it out. Problem the hardest, but tell yourself that it's only temporary. That the feeling will pass.

Using your Triggers

You can also use your triggers for good. Task association is a good way to control your triggers. For instance, doctors have helped insomniacs by telling them to only go to bed when they are sleepy. If they can't sleep, they are told to go to a different room that way their bed is only associated with sleep. This could work to cut back on environmental triggers.

Instead of keeping snacks close to your work area, keep them in the kitchen or break room. That way you associate your desk with working and not with eating. Train yourself to associate your car with singing along with the radio instead of smoking. Only eat at the kitchen table and not on the couch. That way the couch is only for watching TV and the kitchen table is for eating.

CHAPTER FOUR

A SIMPLE BREAK

I'm going to start with the most basic three steps of breaking a bad habit. I don't want to overload you with a bunch of information. These first three basic steps will give you the building blocks to move onto more in-depth information.

The first step you have to take in breaking a habit is the decision to break the habit. You're probably thinking, "Duh," but you have to make sure you have a reason. If you don't have a reason to quit, you will not quit. You won't get anywhere if you go at this thinking you "might" have something you need to change. You have to know and want to change. Make a list of the reasons why you want to stop. If you can't think of anything, make a list of the bad things that will happen if you don't stop. For example, if you don't stop binge eating you could become overweight and develop serious health problems.

The next step is to be ready to face your boredom or emotions. As mentioned before habits are formed out of boredom or stress. You have to be willing to take a look at your life and figure out how to change what is causing your dissatisfaction. You must be ready to face the discomfort. We as humans don't like discomfort, but if you can overcome that, then you have surpassed one of the biggest hurdles. Make your life the way you want it to be.

The last step is to find a new way to relieve stress. You could have the life of your dreams, but you still suffer from stress. You feel stressed, so you turn to alcohol. You drink, and then you don't feel stressed. That makes you think you have everything together. Instead, you need to replace you drinking with something new, something healthy. You could use meditation or exercise as a healthy alternative.

The first three steps are:

1. Make sure you have a good reason to break your habit

2. Be ready to face the emotions and boredom that is causing your habit

3. Find a new way to handle your stress

Starting with these three steps will put you well on your way to breaking your bad habit. In the coming chapters, I will go into more detail on how to switch out your bad habits for new healthy habits.

A Big Break

As learned in the last chapter, there are three necessary steps to breaking habits. While those three steps are paramount there are other tips and tricks to take your habit breaking to the next level. We'll discuss several of them in this chapter, and flesh out even more throughout the rest of the book. A big part of break a bad habit is replacing it with a new one; I'll wait until later to explain how to start said new habit. Now, let's look at some tips to kick those habits to the curb.

1. Set a Start Date

Mark it on your calendar when you want to start changing your habit. You have to be serious about this, so having a countdown will help you to stay on track. The countdown will help to create excitement. Just like a child counting down the 25 to Christmas, or the days before their birthday. You want to drastically change your life for the better, so there should be an element of excitement.

2. Bait and Switch

Once you know what habit you want to change then, you can sub a new habit, temporary or permanent, in its place. If you're a nail-biter, try subbing in gum. Gum can also be used to help with smoking urges.

3. Discover your triggers

Knowing why we make certain decisions is the key to conquering your habits. Often we perform the habit without even realizing we're doing it. That's why it's called a habit. For a long time after my Dad quit smoking, every time he got in the car he would roll down the window and fiddle with his pocket because that's what he would do when he smoked. He never even realized he was doing that until we told him.

But you can fix that by being consciously aware of when you perform your habit. There are five main triggers for habits; location, time, emotional state, other people, and an immediately preceding action. Start to take notes whenever you perform the bad habit. Soon you will be able to figure out what is triggering your problem.

4. Don't go cold turkey

Everybody has probably tried to give up something cold turkey. Cold turkey is a favorite of smokers, but it rarely ever works. It's similar to telling a child to not do something, and that will be exactly what they go and do. Cold turkey is centered on perfection. People think that they if they slip up then they have failed. Nobody is perfect. Cold Turkey leaves no wiggle room, and with something like this, you need a little wiggle room.

5. Switch up your environment

You don't have to move or do anything drastic. The smallest change can switch your brain's thinking. You always smoke in the parking lot at work; the parking lot becomes a trigger. If you change your routine just slightly you will trick your brain into not craving a cigarette. You can also use the 20-second rule. Make it so that it takes 20 more seconds for you to make your habit. If you smoke, keep your cigarettes in a draw where you have to walk to get them. If you have a problem with snacking, put your snacks in the back of the pantry.

6.   Make it incremental

The best way to make a change is to set daily incremental changes. You need to wean yourself off of you habit. The first step is to establish a baseline. This is going to differ according to what you want to change. Such as; how much time you watch TV, how many cigarettes you smoke each day, how many drinks you consume when out with friends. Then choose how much you're going to give up each week. If you're a smoker and you typically smoke a whole pack a day; then the first week or two you go to 15. Then the next two weeks you go down to 10, and so on until you stop smoking.

7.   Don't focus on what you don't want

Most everybody that makes a goal will make this mistake. They will say, I'm not going to do this, or I'm not going to that. Setting a goal like that is setting you up for failure. Instead, decide what you are going to do. It's similar to the bait and switch. If you know you like to snack when working; instead of saying you're not going to snack, say you are going to snack on vegetables. Then all you have to do is switch your chips out for carrots.

8. Do it in honor of yourself

Research shows that people that try to break habits out of frustration or guilt will ultimately fail. People that respect themselves and are happy with who they are will be more successful. Work to change your bad habit from a position of personal strength and confidence.

9. Make a declaration

Social media has become a big part of most everybody's day. Use this to your advantage. Announce on social media the change you are going to make if you feel comfortable doing so. Then keep them updated as you progress. Chances are you will have friends that will congratulate you, and that will make you feel good about what you are doing. This one, of course, isn't for everybody. Some habits that you are trying to break may not be something you want to share with the whole world.

Some habits are very personal, so if you don't feel comfortable sharing it with a large group of people, then you don't have to. Keep in mind though having somebody to talk to can help you along the way.

10. Be prepared to forgive yourself

There will be slip-ups. We are only human beings, and we learn from out slip ups. When you slip up, forgive yourself. Wake up the next day ready to beat your habit. Don't go at it with an all or nothing attitude. There are no scorecards in life. The slip up happened, learn from it, and move on. If you are serious about beating this habit, you won't throw your hands up in defeat after a few lapses.

Classical Conditioning

Classical conditioning is a psychological learning process that occurs when two stimuli are repeatedly paired; a response that is at first elicited by the second stimulus is eventually elicited by the first stimulus alone. An example of this is Pavlov's dog.

Pavlov trained his dog to associate the thrill of being fed with the sound of a bell. He would ring a bell every time he gave the dogs their food. After several repeats of this the dog associated the sound of the bell with receiving food. The dogs would then begin to salivate every time they heard the bell.

This theory doesn't just apply to salivating dogs. Over the years it has formed an important rationale for the development, maintenance, and a relapse of bad habits.

Habits work much in the same way as Pavlov's dogs did. For a smoker, just the site of a pack of cigarettes will elicit a dopamine response causing them to have the urge to smoke. This isn't restricted to smokers either. The same dopamine response happens in alcoholics, overeaters, and so on.

This can be used in reverse, to break a habit. The bell was the trigger for the dogs to start salivating because they knew the food was coming. Just like if a smoker always lights up when they get in the car. The car is the trigger for the smoker to want to smoke. If you start ringing the bell for the dog but don't give them food they will eventually learn that the bell no longer means food. If you stop lighting up every time you get in the car eventually you won't have that trigger anymore.

This is definitely one of the more complicated and harder ways of breaking a habit, but it will work. All the rest have ways of distracting your brain, making it easier to change.

Procrastination

Everybody has been faced with procrastination at some point. It can also be detrimental in your ability to break a habit. But just like breaking a habit, you can overcome procrastination.

In a nutshell, procrastination is when you continually put off doing something. The first step, like with most things, is **realizing you are procrastinating**. If you're honest with yourself, then you know when you are procrastinating, but if you're not sure here are some ways to know;

- Waiting for the right mood, or day to start something

- Doing unimportant tasks to avoid what you need to be doing

- Sitting down to start working, then immediately going to do something else

Once you've realized you are procrastinating, then you can move onto the next step.

Figure out why you are procrastinating. It could be either you or the task. You might find the task unpleasant. Which, since you're changing a habit, you probably will find the task unpleasant. You could also be disorganized or overwhelmed. An important part of the habit breaking process is being organized and knowing what you are doing. Another reason could be that your heart is not into it. You don't have a good enough reason to change this habit.

Lastly, **adopt anti-procrastination strategies**. Procrastination itself is a habit. As you've learned, the only way of getting rid of a habit is persistently not doing the habit. The same tricks you have or will learn about breaking a habit will work to keep you from procrastination. Set up a reward system. Have somebody check in with you. Anything that will keep you accountable in some way, shape, or form.

Be Prepared

Unfortunately, a fact of the world is there will be people that want to sabotage you and your goals. It's not bad enough that you will have self-Sabotaging moments, but you will have to handle other people trying to do the same thing. You have to be prepared to ignore them. They may or may not know what they're doing. Their words can be poison to your success. The moment you start taking their words of "advice" will be your first steps towards failure. Having a plan to handle naysayers is just as important to know what you'll do when you have urges. Make sure you know what to say or do when negative comments arise.

CHAPTER FIVE

A NEW YEAR'S PROBLEM

What's something you get asked every New Year? What's your New Year's resolution? For the first few weeks of the year, every person you see will ask you the same thing. It's expected of everybody to make a New Year's resolution, yet they don't work for people. At least not the way people use them. There's a saying that the definition of insanity is doing the same over and over and again expecting a different result. Then why do people continue to try to make and keep a resolution? People think that resolutions will help them to break some of their bad habits. First, let's look at why a resolution does not work.

1. You're setting the wrong goals.

The most common resolution is to lose weight or get in shape. You wake up the first of January, hop out of bed and say, "I'm going lose 50 pounds this year." By the 15th of January, when you're supposed to be at the gym, you're watching reruns of "The Big Bang Theory" while eating a pint of rocky road. You did nothing wrong. Keeping goals takes more thought than just stating them. These types of goals have little to no leeway. When something happens, and you fail, you will be less likely to make more in the future.

2. Your resolution rarely has to do with the real problem.

You decide to run out and get that gym membership on January first. Good luck fighting the crowd. The gym is going to be packed with everybody else just like you. Once you're in there, you start comparing yourself to everybody. It will definitely help you work through deep-seated psychological issues with inadequacy, rejection, competitiveness and insecurity, but it won't help you solve the real problem. If your goal is to be healthier, then the gym might help, but if you have a problem overeating then it's not going to help. More than likely you're still coming home and eating all the calories you burned off earlier.

3. You set too many.

When making a New Year's resolution a lot of people will think, "While I'm changing this I'll go ahead a change this." Their list of resolutions ends up looking like this;

- Be a better person

- Lose weight

- Sleep more

- Learn a new language

- Drink less

And so on. I get stressed just looking at the list. Our body, as it is, is in homeostasis. It's happy and doesn't want to be changed. The brain has only a finite amount of willpower, and if you start trying to change too many things at once, the brain becomes overwhelmed. The first two weeks of keeping your 10 resolutions may go well, but then your brain starts to smoke and eventually just stops. Then you fall back into old habits.

4. They're too vague.

Let's look at the list above again.

- Be a better person

- Lose weight

- Sleep more

- Learn a new language

- Drink less

They all have something in common. They're about as clear as muddy water. There is no definite way to know if you passed or failed. It's like you teacher gave you an okay on your report card instead of an A or B.

- I want to learn a new language- Great, but what language? Are you trying to learn all languages or a specific one? How are you going to learn your new language? You have no definite plan on how to learn that mysterious new language.

- I want to lose weight- Alright, but how much? Are you overweight and you want to get to a healthier BMI? Do you just want to lose an extra five pounds to fit back into that old dress? You approach those options in very different ways. You have to know how much and why you want to lose weight.

- I want to be a better person- That's admirable, but how? How do you want to be a better person? Do you have a bad temper? Do you use your phone too much? In what way to you want to change? It's great you want to be a better person, but you have to know what aspect of you that you need to change to achieve that goal.

With this new information as to why New Year's resolutions have a tendency to fail, we can now discover how to make them work. No need to swear them off, instead learn how to make them so that you will actually keep them.

1. Be the person you want to be.

The key to keeping any goal is to imagine that you have already achieved your goal. Don't just say, "I'm going to lose weight," or, "I'm going to stop smoking." Be that person. Visualize you eating healthier and working out regularly. Everybody knows the saying "fake it till you make it," this is the same concept. The more you believe on the inside you are already there, the more it will show on the outside.

2. Make them simple.

In fact make them so stupid simple that completing one seems too easy. Remember the acronym KISS, keep it simple stupid. The simpler the goal is, the easier it is to tell that you have accomplished something.

- If you want to drink less hold yourself to drinking one less drink each day, or each week. Then the next week cut out another drink. Continue doing just that, each week, until you reach your overall goal. You'll know you're achieving your goal when you drink less this week than you did the last.

- If you want to sleep more, start setting the alarm to go to bed. If you typically go to bed at midnight, set the alarm on your phone to go off at 10:30 telling you to get ready for bed. That way you will be in bed by eleven. You'll start waking up more refreshed, and you will quickly see that you're achieving your goals.

- If you want to lose weight set your goal to eat more fruits and vegetables each week. Instead of have French fries with your burger have carrot sticks. Start switching out the high-fat sides with whole veggies. You will start seeing a significant change, and you will know you're achieving your goals.

3. Make yourself more accountable.

When people set a resolution, there's nothing that happens to them if they fail, besides the fact that they don't achieve their goal. Instead of having an easy way out, make it painful to not succeed. Dietbet.com is a website that will help you do just that. They have helped over 150,000 people achieve their weight loss goals. The way it works is you choose one of their plans, which you have to pay for. If you achieve your goal, you will win a part of the pot, the money you put in plus some. If you don't achieve your goal, you get nothing. Of course, you don't need their website to do the same thing. If your goal is to quit smoking tell everybody that if you smoke a cigarette, you will pay x amount of dollars to an acquaintance/co-worker/charity that you don't like. Not only are you giving to something or someone you don't like, but you are also spending money that you could use for something you want or need.

4. Keep the number down.

You probably have a million things you want to change, but you have to narrow down your resolution. As I mentioned before your brain only has a finite amount of change willpower. If you deplete it, then you won't achieve anything. Instead make one very simple goal, which is easy to track, and achieve that first. Once you have achieved that goal, and are confident you created a new habit, then start working on another goal.

New Year's resolutions can either help you or hurt you in your habit breaking goal. You have to be extremely careful in the execution. They can be a good way to help you achieve your goals.

CHAPTER SIX

HABIT FORMING

Bad habits. Now we're going to move into a different direction. It's easier, when trying to break a bad habit, to transform it into a good habit. Not only are you eliminating something wrong, you're also forming something good. It's a win-win. Aristotle said, "We are what we repeatedly do. Excellence then is not an act, but a habit." When you were a child learning how to tie your shoes, you had to repeatedly practice over and over again before you learned how. Now you tie your shoes without even thinking. The same goes for forming a new healthy habit.

There are a lot of programs out there that say if you do something for 21 days it will be stuck in your brain. That's true to an extent. Chances are if you have successfully done your goal for 21 days in a row; you will continue to do it. But like all things, it doesn't necessarily work for everybody or every goal. Fulfilling your goal for 21 days is a huge step in the right direction as long as you remember that you still have to actively work to maintain it.

The Three R's

I spoke earlier about the three step structure of forming a habit. You can develop a new habit using that same knowledge. The three R's are; reminder, routine, reward. 'Reminder' is the trigger for your habit. Routine is the habit itself. 'Reward' is the positive thing that makes your brain want to continue to repeat the habit.

Step one is to set a reminder for your new habit. You definitely do need motivation to start a new habit, but motivation isn't enough. And it's definitely not the only way. You have to remember to do your new habit. There are several ways to remind yourself to do something. It could simply be putting your workout clothes someplace where you will see them as soon as you wake up. Set the alarm on your phone telling you to eat a healthy lunch. No matter what it is that you want to start doing, you have to remember to do it.

Picking the right reminder is key, though. The best way I know to figure out when to set a reminder is to make a couple of lists. On the first list write down everything you do every day without fail. For example; brushing your teeth, eating breakfast, going to work, turn off lights, go to bed, and so on. Those are all good things you already do that can remind you to perform your new habit. Such as, after I eat breakfast, I'll go for a walk.

On the second list write down everything that happens to you every day. For example; you stop at a stop sign, you hear your favorite song, a commercial comes on, and you get a text. With both of this list you have a wide array of things that you already respond to that you can use as a reminder. If you want to start moving more, every time you hear your favorite song, dance to it. Don't do this if you're driving, though.

Step two is to create a habit that is super easy to start. There are lots of shows on TV showing people shedding lots of weight in a short amount of time. Or you see the runners or swimmers at the Olympics. It makes you want to achieve the same thing. Everybody has those moments where you think you can be just like them. The enthusiasm is great, but it's important to know that lasting changes are a product of habit. Remember, in the words of Leo Babauta, "Make it so easy that you can't say no." At first, performance doesn't matter. The only thing that matters is you strive to do something. Don't worry about how long you run, or how many veggies you eat, it just matters that you are running or eating vegetables. First, decide what you want your new habit to be. Then ask yourself, "How can I make this so easy that I can't say no?"

Step three is to create a reward. You have to celebrate. Celebration is an important part of life. You want to continue to do something that makes you feel good. Since you have to repeat an action for it to become a habit you have to find a way to reward yourself for doing it. If your goal is to exercise, then every time you finish a work out tell yourself, "Good job," or, "Today was a great day." You can also choose to say "Victory" or "Success" every time you practice the new habit. Give yourself credit no matter how big or small the success was.

Step by Step

That's an easy way to start adopting a new healthy habit. Some habits are going to be harder than others to adopt. Here are few other tips to help adopt a new habit.

Make the habit daily. New habits that you only do every few days are harder to adopt. If you want to start exercising, make sure you exercise once a day for the first 30 days. After the first 30 days, you can step down to three or four times a week.

Write down your goal. When you write out, with pen and paper, what you want your goal to be, it will make it seem more important. It makes your idea more real when you write it down.

Make it so you can't lose. Tell yourself you're running an experiment. You're running an experiment for 30 days by doing this new habit. Experiments can't fail. It makes it seem a lot less stressful. Nothing matters until after the first 30 days, and by that time you have adopted your new habit.

A big downfall of people adopting a new habit is that they doubt there self. When you first start working out you may have the thought, "I can't do this as well as they can." Whenever that thought pops into your head add, "But if I continue to work out I will get better at it." You can use this technique with anything.

Know what could happen. Be sure you know all the consequences of not starting your new habit, and know the impact of starting your new habit. Suppose your goal is eating healthier. If you don't start eating healthier, you could start gaining weight and develop health problems. If you do start eating healthier, you will lose weight and have more energy during the day.

Do it for yourself. Don't bog yourself down with the thoughts of what you should do. Instead, focus on what you want to do. You're making these changes for yourself and not for anybody else. Work towards things that motivate you and make your life better. Don't think you have to live your life like everybody around you does.

Switch Bad for Good

One of the best ways to break a bad habit is to switch it out for a good one. It helps to trick your brain and contributes to reduce cravings.

- As always, you have to first identify your triggers. You cannot break bad habits until you figure out what triggers them.

- For every trigger identify a good habit that you could do instead. Instead of smoking when you wake up, what are you going to do? Good habits could be; exercise, meditation, decluttering, organizing, and more.

- For, at least a month, be consistent with those triggers. Every time a trigger comes up act on the good habit you decided to do. The more consistent you are, the more the new habit will become ingrained, and the less you will think of the bad habit.

- Avoid severe trigger situations. You can't always switch out all triggers for new habits. As mentioned before, you might want to skip going out with friends after work for a little while. At least until you get a handle on controlling your urges.

- Discover ways to fight the strong urges. Even though the goal is to switch out the bad habit for a good habit, you will still get the urge to do the bad habit. You will likely need a backup plan when fighting urges.

- Find supportive help. Have somebody you can talk to if things get really rough. Some bad habits are tougher to break than others, and you will go through some tough times, so having somebody you can talk to will help you work through the tough times.

- Stay positive. There will be times when negative thoughts pop into your head. You will have self-sabotaging moments. But the key is to stay positive. When negative thoughts come up, remind yourself why you're doing this. Remind yourself that you're changing yourself for the better.

CHAPTER SEVEN

BE SUPPORTIVE

The human mind has the amazing ability to be able to talk you out of doing what you know is right. It can come up with crazy reasons why you shouldn't do something that you know you need to do. You want to work out, "Why? It will make you sweaty." You want to quit smoking, "You'll feel more stress if you do." You want to go to be earlier, "But then you'll miss Jimmy Kimmel." See what I mean. You have to find a way to tell your brain to shut up, and an accountability partner will help you do just that.

Growing up you probably had friends that you would vent to, and they would help you feel better about a situation. An accountability partner works much in the same way.

It will probably feel foreign or uncomfortable the first time. That's a good thing. The uncomfortable feeling is your brain resisting the change. Embrace those feelings. It will be worth it once you work through them.

The role of an accountability partner is to keep you accountable. They help as an outside force to tell your brain to shut up. Their only purpose is to keep you on track. They are there for you when you feel like straying from your path. They're there for you when you wake up in the middle of the night wanting a cupcake. Or when you are extremely stressed out, and you want a cigarette.

Your partner can be anybody that you resonate with. There is no need to pay a professional. They could be a family member, co-worker, friend, or somebody else that is trying to achieve the same goal. Find someone that you connect with and trust to hold you accountable. Be completely open about your goal. What you want to achieve and when you want to achieve it. They are there to be your cheerleader and to hold you to your commitment. Here are some things to look for in choosing your accountability partner:

1. They're reliable. They are easily reached whenever wherever.

2. They want to be your partner. You can't make somebody help you, so make sure they actually want to.

3. Make sure they can relate to you in some way. You don't want to pick someone that has never tried to lose weight to help you lose weight. They won't understand what you're going through.

4. You feel comfortable being honest and open with them, and they are comfortable giving you honest feedback.

Now that you know how to pick your accountability partner, let's talk about the benefits they will provide you. One of the biggest benefits to having an accountability partner is they will accelerate your performance. When you connect with someone one-on-one, you are able to work through the problems of your plan with them. You'll be able to make a sure fire plan to achieve your goals.

Your partner will help you measure your achievements. A good partner will help you to set milestones to reach along the way. It will be easier for you to keep track of your success, and keep you from becoming discouraged. Their outside eyes will see your success more easily than you will be able to.

They will help to validate your thoughts and ideas. Having someone to bounce your ideas off of, besides yourself, will help you to make decisions. They can give you honest outside information. They will help to silence your inner critic.

They help to keep you engaged. Things will come up that will try to distract you from your goals, and you will have someone there to help you stay the path. When you're bored, they will be there for you to talk to. Just knowing that you have somebody there for you will help you to keep your eye on the prize.

Ultimately they will hold you responsible. They are there behind you, pushing you towards your goals. They keep you from getting distracted and hold you accountable. Having a weekly check in with someone, and knowing you have to tell them what you have done this week to achieve your goal, will make you more likely to stay proactive. They keep you from making excuses, and, instead, make deliberate actions towards your end goal.

This isn't to say that you can't achieve your goals by yourself. There are people out there that can, but it takes a lot more willpower. Having a support system will make all the difference in the world.

CHAPTER EIGHT

BOOST YOUR POWER

And that's willpower. Willpower is probably one of the last things you need to work on though. If you don't know what you're trying to change, or why you're doing it, then willpower isn't going to help. You could have great willpower, but without a purpose it's going to fall flat. It's like building a house. You can have all the wood you need, but if you don't have the nails, it's not going to stay together. Once you have your plan in place, then you can move onto willpower.

Willpower and self-control are imperative building blocks for a happy and prosperous life. Some of the most persuasive evidence comes from these two studies.

The first is the marshmallow experiment. Psychologist Walter Mischel started the experiment in the 1960s. He would offer four-year-olds a choice of a marshmallow now or two marshmallows if they could wait 15 minutes. He and his associates then tracked those students as they grew up. They found that the children who were willing to wait 15 minutes for the marshmallows achieved greater academic success, better health, and a less likely chance of divorce.

In the second study, 1,000 children were studied from birth to 32. Researchers found that the children's self-control could predict the future of their health, substance dependence, criminal offenses, and personal finances. It was even true when they eliminated factors such as intelligence and social class.

Use it or lose it

Everybody knows these two factors about muscles:

- Muscles get stronger when exercised

- Muscles can be overworked, which leaves them weak until they have time to rest

But here are some interesting things you may not know.

- In a study, some participants were told not to think about a white bear. Thought-suppression takes a good deal of self-control, especially when told not to think about something. After that, they were told to limit their intake of beer during a taste test because there would be a driving test later. The thought-suppression participants drank more than the non-thought-suppression participants.

- In another study, participants that were asked to suppress their emotions during an upsetting movie gave up sooner during a physical stamina test than those who were freely allowed to express their emotions.

- In a third study, women watched a documentary while seated near a candy bowl. In some, the candy bowl was right next to the woman, in others the candy bowl was across the room from them. Later, they were given hard puzzles to solve. Those that had been seated close to the candy bowl gave up sooner than those who weren't.

In each of these studies, the people that were forced to overuse their willpower or self-control could not fully finish subsequent tasks. Their willpower had been depleted. Now let's look at some ways to strengthen your willpower.

1.   Don't keep your willpower depleted

If you have plans to help your friend move heavy pieces of furniture, you're not going to spend 30 minutes before lifting weights. You know your energy will be depleted before you help your friend. The same goes for your willpower. Exercising self-control is an excellent way to build willpower, never giving yourself a break is a good way to deplete it.

2.   Meditation

Meditation seems to come up a lot when looking for ways to change habits. It is a great way to strengthen your ability to control your thoughts. But what is meditation? Meditation is simply the practice of bringing your thoughts to the present moment. 47% of lives are spent either thinking about the past, or what has to be done in the future. Leaving us with very little time to think about what we are doing at this present moment. Our brains are very undisciplined. They like to wander. With 10 minutes of meditation each day it will help strengthen your mind and help keep it from wandering. Studies have shown after just 2 to 3 days of 10-minute meditation your brain will be able to focus better, you will have more energy and a lot less stress.

3. Use your imagination

Imagination is an amazing way to improve willpower. The body can respond the same way to an imaginary scenario as the real one. If you imagine laying on a beach, listening to the waves crash, your body will respond by relaxing. On the other hand, if you think about going to work and having a meeting with your boss, your body will tense in response. Dieters are in a constant state of depletion. As a result, they feel everything more intensely. Imagination is able to help control these irritations

In a study, participants were asked to watch a movie with a bowl of chocolate placed nearby. One group was told to imagine they had decided to eat as much as they want. The second group was told to imagine they had eaten none. The third group was told to imagine they had decided to eat the chocolate later. The first group ate more than the other two. Then when given the opportunity to eat later, those that had imagined they would eat later, ate less than the others. They even reported a lesser desire to consume the candy.

4. Use your opposite hand

Researchers have conducted studies that tested corrective actions. One they found that worked particularly well was to use your opposite hand. Your brain is wired to use your dominant hand so it will take willpower to use the non-dominate hand. To practice this, choose a time during the day to use your non-dominate hand. I would suggest doing no more than an hour at a time. More than an hour may deplete your willpower

5. Distract yourself

It's even possible to use your imagination to distract yourself from unwanted thoughts. Just like in the study mentioned earlier about the white bear. When you tell yourself not to think about something, it's going to continually pop back into your head. Train yourself to think about something else. If you don't want to think about that white bear, or cigarettes, or candy, flip your thoughts to something else. Instead of a white bear, think of a black bear. Instead of cigarettes, think of chewing gum. Instead of candy, think of fruit. That puts you in complete control of your thoughts

6. Control your stress

I have mentioned stress several times throughout this book. Stress is the main culprit of many problems. When you become stressed, you'll tend to fall back into old habits. Most of the time you won't even realize it because your body goes into autopilot. When you're stressed, your body releases stress hormones, mainly cortisol.

Cortisol increases your cravings for carbohydrates. Carbs will lower your cortisol levels. Which is probably perhaps why you turn to your friends Ben and Jerry. Alcohol is also a depressant that reduces your cortisol levels. Both of those options hold some negative side effect and aren't helping you to kick those bad habits.

Fortunately, we know these things so you can have control over what you do. The stress response is the same as the fight or flight response, so anything that counterattacks that response will do. Start responding to those stressors by listening to calming music, visualizing calming scenes, or moderate exercise. Whatever works for you. Researchers also say viewing funny videos can help counteract willpower depletion.

The more you practice these habits, the more likely they will be there to help you when major stressors arise.

7. A step at a time

Most of the time people give up on goals, not because of the lack of willpower, but because of feeling overwhelmed in what they are trying to accomplish. I have mentioned something similar to this before. Break your goals down into manageable pieces. That way you can see each step you take instead of trying to consume the whole thing. This also keeps you from depleting your willpower, keeping you recharged and ready to continue working at all times.

8. Be yourself

It takes a lot of effort to suppress you typical behaviors, personality, and preferences. Not surprisingly, it also depletes willpower. Psychologist Mark Muraven found that people who exert self-control to make others happy were more easily depleted than individuals who held true to their own goals and happiness. People pleasures may find they are at a disadvantage when it comes to willpower as opposed to those who are secure and comfortable with their self.

9. Change your speech

In another correction study, researchers conducted to modify the subject's natural speech. This would include resisting the urge to say a cuss word, or simply change from saying "hey" to "hello." It takes willpower to make the conscious effort to change one's speech, especially when we typically speak out of instinct. It doesn't matter what you do to change your speech, as long as you make a conscious effort to switch things up. Just like using your opposite hand, choose a chunk of your day where you will change the way you speak. You also need to decide what it is that you are going to change. You might choose to stop swearing, or to stop saying slang words like "ain't." Remember to only practice this for about an hour at a time, or you may deplete your willpower. After only two weeks you will see an increase in your willpower.

10. Keep temptations at bay

With most habits, you have a weakness for what you like to consume. If you drink too much keep alcohol out of your house. If you smoke, get rid of all your cigarettes. If you snack a lot, either get rid of the junk food or put it out of sight. There will be times when you see your weakness, and you will need to make a plan for that moment. Decide how you are going to handle it. If your weakness is junk food and you have children, chances are junk food is going to enter your house at some point. No matter where the kids got the food, grandma, trick or treating, school, work out a plan where you don't constantly see it. Work with your spouse or significant other. Have them take all the junk food and put it where you don't know where it is. If the kids want some, they have to ask the other parent, not you. And you have to promise that you won't beg and plead to know where it is. That takes a little willpower in itself, but a lot less than trying to keep from eating the junk food that you see.

Willpower is just like any other muscle in your body. With the right practice, it can be strengthened. I have just given you 10 ways to increase your willpower and self-control, but don't try to do all 10 at once. You'll just end up driving yourself crazy. Think of training your willpower just like you would prepare for a race. On your first day of training, you're not going to run the full 26 miles. Not unless you're already an Olympic runner. Instead, you will increase the amount you run every day. Choose one of these to start using on a daily basis. Once you feel that's not working for you anymore, pick a different one. Before you know it, you will be more mentally strong.

CHAPTER NINE

MEDITATIVE STATE

Mediation has proved to be very helpful in most aspects of life. It has shown up numerous times already in this book. Since it seems to be so useful, I figured I would dedicate a whole chapter to it. We'll take a deeper look into the benefits of meditation and how it will help you break your bad habits. Then I will give you a simple step by step on how to get started meditating for beginners. If you already meditate, then you have a leg up.

Ask anybody that meditates, and they will tell you it's good for you. But in what way? Is that just from years of practice, or is there scientific research out there that proves it's good for you? Here are some general ways that mediation can help:

- Improves willpower

- Improves focus

- Decreases stress

- Improves ability to learn

- Increases energy

There are over 3,000 scientific studies that examine the benefits of meditation. I'm going to summarize some of the findings for you.

- Decreases depression

In Belgium, a study was conducted at five middle schools involving approximately 400 students. Professor Filip Raes concluded that the students that participated in mindfulness meditation reduced indication of anxiety, stress, and depression for up to six months later. At the University of California, a similar study was conducted with formerly depressive patients and concluded that mindfulness meditation reduced ruminative thinking and dysfunctional beliefs.

- Reduces panic disorder

The American Journal of Psychiatry published a study where 22 patients diagnosed with panic disorder were submitted to 3 months of meditation and relaxation training. 20 of the 22 participants showed that their panic and anxiety had been reduced significantly, and the changes were maintained at follow-up.

- Increases concentration

Harvard neuroscientists ran an experiment where 16 people took part in an 8-week mindfulness course. They used guided meditation and integration of mindfulness in everyday activities. Sara Lazer, Ph.D., reported at the end, MRI scans showed that gray matter concentration increased in areas of the brain involved in learning, memory, emotion regulation, sense of self, and perspective.

- Increases focus in spite of distraction

Emory University did a study that demonstrated that participants with more mediation experience exhibited increased connectivity within the brain controlling attention. The neural relationships may be involved in the development of cognitive skills.

- Prevents you from falling in a multitasking trap

Multitasking is a dangerous productivity myth that will deplete you of energy and is a source of stress. Switching between tasks is costly to your brain which can cause feelings of distraction and dissatisfaction. In a study conducted by the University of Washington and the University of Arizona, human resources personnel took part in 8 weeks of in either mindfulness meditation or body relaxation techniques. They were given stressful multitasking tests before and after training. Groups that had practice meditation showed lower stress levels and a better recall of the tasks they had done. They also switched between tasks less often, concentrating on one task for a longer amount of time.

- Increases unconscious mind awareness

A study done by the University of Sussex found that people who practiced mindfulness meditation experienced a longer paused between unconscious impulses and action. They were also less susceptible to hypnosis.

- Reduces heart diseases and stroke

Cardiovascular disease kills more people in the world than anything else. A study performed in 2012, studied 200 high-risk individuals. They were asked to, either, take part in a health education class promoting better diet and exercise, or take a class on transcendental meditation. During the next five years, they found that those who took the meditation class decreased their overall risk of heart disease, stroke, and death by 48%.

- Increases compassion and decreases worry

After 9 weeks of compassion cultivation training, participants showed significant improvement in all three domains of compassion (compassion for others, receiving compassion, and self-compassion).

- Decreases emotional eating

Scientists have found that transcendental meditation decreases the likelihood of emotional eating, which helps to prevent obesity.

There is a lot more scientific information out there that proves meditation can help with all aspects of life. It's no wonder that it shows up a lot in contributing to quit bad habits.

Simple meditation practice

If you've never meditated before, I would suggest doing a guided meditation. A quick search on the internet will turn up several apps and downloads for guided meditation. Some free choices are Omvana, Headspace, Calm, Smiling Mind, and Take a Break.

If you want to meditate on your own here is a simple meditation practice designed by Headspace App founder, Andy Puddicombe:

1. Find a quiet room where you can sit comfortably upright with no distraction.

2. Set a 10-minute timer, and get comfortable in your chair.

3. Find something in your line of vision to focus on for 6 deep breaths. With each exhale, allow your body to soften as you become more relaxed. On the 6th exhale, close your eyes.

4. Focus your attention on the points of contact between your body and the chair and floor. Notice the sensation of your arms, back, and bottom on the chair, and your feet on the floor.

5. Then become aware of your surroundings. Notice all the sounds and smells around you. Anything that you can sense without your sight.

6. Then focus on your breath. Notice how your chest expands when you breathe in and how it contracts when you exhale.

7. Once you're comfortable with the rhythm of your breathing, begin to count. 1 on the inhale, 2 on the exhale, all the way up to 10. This will keep your mind focused on your breath and keep it from wandering.

8. When you make it to 10, start back over at 1. Do not count 11, 12, 13, etc.

9. While you breathe, allow your thoughts to come and go. You can't stop yourself from thinking. What you want to do is avoid lingering on one thought. The moment you realize your mind has wandered, bring it back to your breaths.

10. Continue until your timer goes off.

The first time you do this, it will probably seem awkward and weird. It's just like adopting a new habit. The more you do it, the less uncomfortable it becomes, and the easier it will be to do.

Here are some other, more advanced, mediation options:

- Candle starting

If you have problems focusing, you can light a candle and stare at it. Make sure the candle is at eye level. If you find your mind wandering, return your focus to what the flame is doing. Another level up is to stare at the candle without blinking. It will eventually make you cry which refreshes your eyes.

- Mantra

The repetition of words helps you to find calm and focus. You can find different mantras online, or you can make up your own. It doesn't matter what you say as long as it resonates with you, and you're happy with it.

- Visualization

Another fun and easy way to meditate is to visualize an idyllic being or setting in your mind. You can make it whatever you want. Embellishing it as much or as little as you need.

- Become the Observer

Become the observer of your mind. Close your eyes and focus on the spot, about an inch, above the spot between your eyebrows, third eye chakra. Begin to focus on what you mind and body is feeling, thinking and doing.

You should now be able to use meditation to help you break your bad habits, and, in the process, start a new good, habit.

I'm sure you are dying to start working on getting rid of that bad habit that's been bothering you, so I'll wrap this up. Remember to keep this simple. Don't overwhelm yourself with too many goals, or trying too many of these techniques at once. Be prepared to fail and meet naysayers, they are inevitable, but you don't have to let them control you. If nothing else, please remember you deserve to live the best life possible.

CPSIA information can be obtained
at www.ICGtesting.com
Printed in the USA
LVHW010026150121
676462LV00005B/761

9 789814 952170